The
Dog Lover's Guide
to Massage

What Your Dog Wants You to Know

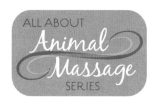

The Dog Lover's Guide to Massage

What Your Dog Wants You to Know

Megan Ayrault, LMP, L/SAMP

Licensed Massage Practitioner
Large and Small Animal Massage Practitioner

www.AllAboutAnimalMassage.com

This book is intended for animal owners and caregivers to learn information and skills that will complement care from professionals, including from veterinarians. It is not intended as a substitute for veterinary advice, diagnosis, or treatment. Animal owners should consult their veterinarians regularly, including in regard to any symptoms that may require diagnosis or treatment.

Any animal handling, including massage and bodywork, holds the potential for harm to handler, animal or both. The author and her associates offer important safety guidelines, but assume no liability for how the information in this book, or in the other resources at AllAboutAnimalMassage.com, is implemented.

Published by
All About Animal Massage
PO Box 56, Kirkland, Washington 98083
www.AllAboutAnimalMassage.com

First Edition

Edited and packaged by CeciBooks Editorial & Publishing
Cover and interior design by Karen Johnson, Level 29 Design
Photographs by Ann Chase Photography
Illustrations by Margo McKnight, ©The Northwest School of Animal Massage

Library of Congress Cataloging-in-Publication Data
Ayrault, Megan
The dog lover's guide to massage: what your dog wants you to know / by Megan Ayrault.
ISBN: 978-0-9822556-0-5

1. Dogs—Disease—Alternative Treatment 2. Animal Massage 3. Complementary Care 4. Title

Dedication

If you love someone,
the greatest gift you can give them
is your true presence.

Thich Nhat Hanh

Our animals generously offer us this gift every day. How often do we truly receive it? Or return it? Could we learn to do better?

This seemingly simple act of offering our true presence, as well as receiving another's, is at the heart of all bodywork, including massage.

I'm grateful to my many animal and human teachers, including colleagues, clients, students, friends, and family. Your support has been generous in many ways, and you continue to teach me about true presence every day. It is a vital lesson, among many, in the art and science of doing bodywork; one that I will always appreciate opportunities to practice.

Contents

Introduction

This book is about more than just dog massage. True, it is about their bodies, and specifically the many ways they respond to massage. More importantly though, it is about deepening your connectedness with the dogs in your life by learning more about what is going on under their skin, and discovering the powerful tool of massage for their physical and emotional health. The process of learning to better care for our animals is never-ending, and this book, along with my other books and website, *www.AllAboutAnimalMassage.com*, is intended to be an important part of that process for you. I also hope that through your love for dogs and your motivation to learn more about caring for them, you will learn more about how your own body works (because it's much the same), and how to better care for yourself as well. As you read this book you will find information, therapeutic techniques, insights, resources, and inspiration for all of these purposes.

Massage for people and now also for animals is becoming more mainstream every passing year as the many benefits are experienced and recognized. Dog owners everywhere are learning how massage and bodywork can contribute significantly to ease of movement, health, and quality of life for their dogs. Of course this is in addition to the regular care from your dog's veterinarian. After reading this book you will not only be able to massage your dog, but you will understand exactly what each technique is doing, how the body is benefiting, and how massage works.

Part one of this book, "A Consumer's Guide to Dog Massage," focuses on two topics. The first and most fascinating one is how your dog's body responds to outside influences, whether adapting to the effects of stress and trauma or healing in response to massage and bodywork. This information will give you new and deeper insights into what's going on under your dog's skin, which will enhance your awareness of your dog's needs and the effectiveness of your massage. The second focus is professional massage; it provides information that can help you find and work with an animal massage therapist or bodyworker to support your dog's optimal health and well-being. Both topics together will make you a more savvy and educated receiver of massage, whether for your dog or for yourself.

Part two is the how-to portion, "Massaging Your Dog." You will learn massage techniques that will help you monitor, support, and learn about your dog's body. To help you continue to expand your skills further, I have included suggestions on variations of the techniques, and coaching tips to make the quality of your touch more therapeutic as you practice over time. Along with each technique, you will also learn something about your dog's anatomy that relates to that technique. You can use this anatomy information to help you visualize and focus as you massage, enhancing the results for your dog and the fun for yourself.

Parts one and two of this book are designed to work synergistically. That is, by reading either part alone you will learn a lot and help your dog, but if you read and use both parts together, the effect will be more than double. In addition to being a great resource on its own, this book is also part of a larger whole. It is interconnected with its partner website, *www. AllAboutAnimalMassage.com*, where you will find many additional resources, including a panel of Expert Advisors, the free "All About Animal Massage" newsletter, articles, videos, photos, e-books, shared stories and testimonials, training, recommended books, DVDs and other products, and links to further resources, all to continue your education and inspiration into the future. Another great tool here is the "Animal Wellness Network," where animal lovers of all backgrounds and levels of expertise can find, support, and learn from each other for the benefit of all animals. Whether or not you choose to actively participate and create your own profile in this network, you can always use it to search for animal care professionals near you, including massage and bodywork professionals.

Among many books available in the website's store is this book's companion e-book *Massaging My Dog: A Guided Journal*, an interactive workbook that will lead you through the learning process of "Massaging Your Dog," part two of this book.

The journal includes:

• Additional instruction on assessing your dog's body and reading feedback

• Charts and instructions to record your massages

Completing the journal and the charts will help you identify patterns of tension in your dog's body and show the progress you both make together over time.

These guided journals make ideal educational projects for young people, too, including those involved with organizations such as 4-H or Scouts.

For any horse lovers you know (perhaps yourself?), *The Horse Lover's Guide to Massage: What Your Horse Wants You to Know* is a valuable addition to their horse library. Most of the techniques and anatomy taught in *The Horse Lover's Guide* are different from what you will find here for dogs, yet the information can be easily adapted to the other species with a few adjustments.

If you don't have a need for the horse book yourself, you can still get the additional massage techniques and anatomy information by purchasing the supplemental e-book, *More Massage Moves for Dog Lovers*, which contains the techniques and anatomy taught in *The Horse Lover's Guide* already adapted for dogs.

Finally, you will find on the website the free e-book *Animal Massage: A Consumer Guide*, which is similar to but less extensive than part one of this book. It also includes a few things this book does not, so I hope you will take a look at it for yourself, and also refer other animal lovers to it for an easy, accessible, and free introduction to animal massage.

Part One

A Consumer's Guide to Dog Massage

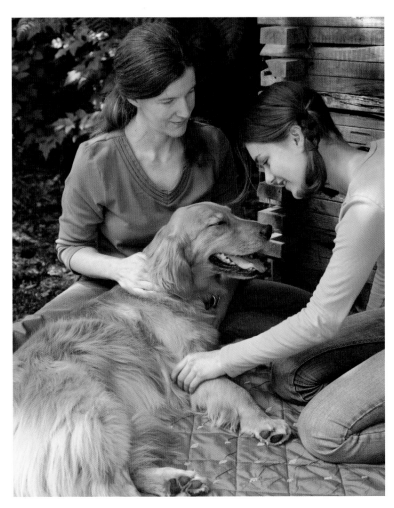

It's easy to provide your dog with many of the benefits massage has to offer.

I

Loving Your Dog with Massage: The Benefits

Picture a puppy at play. See in your mind's eye how fully her whole body participates in every movement. What are some words that come to mind? Joy, energy, exuberance, fluidity, ease, fun!

Now picture the same dog a bit older, then much older. What are the qualities of that movement? Of course, the inner spirit may still share all the qualities described above and more, but for now, just consider how she is moving. How do you sense she is feeling physically? Is it really only age that's making the difference?

Perhaps you know of an older person who is devoted to an activity such as dance, yoga, or a martial art—an activity that promotes both strength and flexibility equally throughout the whole body. How does this person move? Do words like ease, fluidity, and joy come to mind more easily than when you visualized the older dog?

Well, this book is about massage, not dance, yoga, or martial arts, but what do they have in common? Health and vitality, or in other words, joy, energy, exuberance, fluidity, ease, and fun. A lifetime of healthy exercise would certainly promote all of these, but most of our dogs, like most of us, spend too much time not moving much at all, moving in limited, habitual patterns, or moving in ways that are more stressful to the body than healthful. Fortunately, there is another means of creating some of the same benefits that exercise gives us, as well as a few additional ones: massage! Massage does far more than ease sore muscles. What is actually going on under the skin? How is the body responding and changing?

We all know that massage relieves sore muscles and provides some well-deserved pampering. Here are some examples of additional benefits received from massage.

- Boosts the immune system

- Improves the quality and symmetry of movement

- Balances muscle tone for better joint health and function

- Promotes earlier detection of stresses and strains

- Stimulates circulation for greater health of all tissues

- Helps reduce risk, severity, and frequency of injuries

- Improves athletic agility and coordination

- Promotes strength and endurance

- Reduces the effects of stress

- Minimizes restrictions caused by old scar tissue

- Promotes the development of more functional scar tissue during healing

- Reduces or eliminates adhesions, knots, and other restrictions

- Improves skeletal alignment and posture for more efficient movement

- Releases endorphins (natural "feel good" painkillers)

- Lowers blood pressure

- Improves digestion

- Supports recovery from injury, surgery, or other traumas

- Reduces swelling

- Optimizes the training and learning progress due to better health, calmer mind, and greater body awareness and comfort

- Improves the quality of sleep

- Releases stored toxins

- Increases flexibility and resilience

- Deepens your relationship with your animal

How does massage do all that, you might ask? In chapter 3 you will learn six concepts about *how* bodies work, your dog's and your own. Each concept will be explained in a way that shows clearly how various types of bodywork and massage can lead to these significant benefits. That is, any one of the six could be all it takes to make you say, "Wow, massage is cool!" but I'll go through all six anyway to further enlighten you. That way you will also have a good sense of why so many different types of massage all work, just in different ways. You will also see that even if a massage session does not provide the specific result you were looking for, that doesn't mean nothing therapeutic happened.

In fact, this brings me to an important point about understanding the benefits of massage. Some benefits, such as "improves the quality and symmetry of movement," can often be readily seen following a massage, but let's take an example like "helps reduce risk, severity, and frequency of injuries." It can be difficult at best to prove results such as this one because you can't know how your dog would have fared had she *not* received a massage. Let's say you have a professional massage for your dog, and a few days or weeks later she's limping.

Does that mean the massage did no good? Not at all. Perhaps rather than a torn muscle, for example, your dog has now only strained it, possibly thanks to the massage having reduced at least some of the stresses that had been building over time.

We can't prove or disprove such scenarios, but what we can do is look at the physiology of the muscles and other soft tissues; that is, how they work and how massage affects them. Muscles, tendons, and ligaments, for example, are all more prone to injury when muscles are fatigued. Muscles are more prone to fatigue when they are chronically tight and the tissue becomes less resilient, which can happen for many reasons, as discussed in chapter 2. Chapters 3 and 4 will give you information on how the body responds both to stress and to massage, which will better enable you to understand the many benefits of massage. And if you visit *www.AllAboutAnimalMassage.com*, you will find shared stories and observations about the results of massage and bodywork that people have witnessed in their animal companions.

How Does Massage Resemble Car Maintenance?

In this section I'm going to use a machine analogy for the body, but please don't take this to mean that bodies are actually very machine-like. They most definitely are not, neither ours nor our dogs. Too bad for our cars. If they were more like our animals, maybe they could also adapt and compensate, limping along at least enough to get us to the service station when something goes wrong. Wouldn't that be helpful?

Even though living bodies are much more than merely complicated machines, there is one comparison that relates very well to massage. Car maintenance. The idea that sometimes it's wise to take action to prevent a problem, rather than waiting until something breaks down. Yes, you can definitely save money in the short run by not getting oil changes, or new tires, filters, brake pads, etc. But is that really smart? Of course, even if you get the regular service, there's no guarantee your car won't eventually have a problem, but it is likely that over the lifetime of your car you will have fewer and less costly repairs if you invest in maintenance.

So what is optimal for maintenance for your dog's body? Even a car's performance is not totally predictable, let alone a living body's. But you can figure that certain factors will influence how much maintenance a car requires, and also what the odds are that it may also need repairs sooner than later. For a car, these factors include mileage, types of road surfaces, speeds driven, accidents, quality of fuel, condition of tires, and of course the quality of the car to start with (conformation), not to mention whether it's being used for the type of driving for which it was actually designed.

See anything in this list you recognize for your dog? I hope you also see that this analogy applies not only to massage but also to how a dog is exercised and handled, the quality of food, conformation, regular veterinary care of course, and so on. The more challenges your dog has to her body, the more massage can support her.

In this car maintenance analogy, waiting until your dog is injured or obviously in pain before using massage is like waiting for your car to break down in traffic before you ever take it to a mechanic. One significant difference, though, is that your dog is a living being that has been experiencing, except in cases of sudden injury or illness, a gradual onset of symptoms while you were either waiting for them to go away or not paying attention. I know I've made this mistake myself with my own dogs, and I'm a massage therapist!

My point is not to add to any feelings of guilt but just to offer an important reminder for our dogs' sakes. Learning the information in this book will raise the bar of your responsibility to your animals, but only because it will also raise your awareness and your skills to detect the needs of your dog's body sooner than you have been able to in the past. To get back to our analogy, this is just like the way a more experienced and knowledgeable driver is more able and likely to notice early warning signs of trouble in a car's engine, and provide the appropriate care right away.

As you may have already noticed, I sometimes refer to "bodywork" instead of always using the term massage. While the many varieties of massage are types of bodywork, not all bodywork is massage. Here are just a few examples to illustrate the range of bodywork. It can include Sports Massage, Lymphatic Facilitation, Deep Tissue Massage, Acupressure, Shiatsu, Myofascial Release, Craniosacral Therapy, Structural Integration, Rolfing, Trigger Point Therapy, Neuromuscular Therapy, Reflexology, and many, many more. Not to mention new ones being developed almost every day, it seems! Modalities (types of bodywork) may focus on muscles, skeletal alignment, internal organs, the rhythm and flow of cerebral-spinal fluid, the balance of Chi energy in meridian pathways, the stimulation of the lymphatic system, and so on. The information in this book, though its focus is massage, applies to virtually all forms of bodywork. This is because it's about the body, and about various effects therapeutic touch can have on the body, and how those effects happen. You can find out more about varieties of massage and bodywork, or a specific modality, at *www.AllAboutAnimalMassage.com*.

2

Why and When Dogs Need Massage

Dogs in our society often experience phenomenal support, care, and love in many ways. The growing interest in complementary services like massage is a wonderful testimonial to this fact. Yet all dogs, even the same ones we go to great lengths to care for, also face certain challenges to their health and comfort.

As you read the following examples of stress factors for dogs, imagine how each situation might be impacting your own dog's body and health. When you read the next chapter, "How Massage Works," you will find information about your dog's physiology (that is, how the body functions) that will give you more ideas and clearer pictures of what is going on under the skin, first in response to stress, and then in response to massage.

Stress Factors

Lack of movement: This may be due to confinement in a kennel or crate, or it may be just not having enough space to run. Many dogs, even if they do have freedom to move, may choose to nap all day due to boredom, stiffness, or low energy. Some breeds and individuals are also more inclined to "conserve energy" than others.

Injuries: Repetitive stress injuries and trauma are the main categories. Causes can include rough and tumble play, jumping in and out of cars or on and off furniture, falls or other accidents, and prolonged running on hard surfaces. Keep in mind that any surgery can certainly be counted as a trauma from which your dog must heal, even if the surgery had a positive outcome. However an injury occurs, it brings on a cascade of additional stresses to deal with, including the rest of the body having to compensate for the injured area in order to protect it. Often the hours spent confined will be increased and any exercise decreased. Pain and confinement will both make sleep less restful. Medications may stress the organs in a variety of ways.

Pulls on leashes: These pressures may be initiated by either the dog or a human, but either way the dog's body will have forces to resist; the neck being especially vulnerable to developing problems. Intense or sudden pulls (jerks) can obviously cause an injury, but even subtle pressures will have cumulative effects over time. In either case, injury may or may not be obvious right away, but can easily result in problems days, weeks, or even years later. It's very important for the long-term health of a dog's body that he learn not to pull on leashes, whether with traditional or other types of neck collars, head collars, or harnesses.

Genetic weaknesses: Just a few examples that affect the musculo-skelatal system in particular include conformation that makes some dogs or entire breeds more prone to hip dysplasia and luxating patellas (locking kneecaps), and disk (back) problems. Genetic issues can also affect circulation, respiration, the nervous system, and so on. All of these issues can obtain benefits from massage.

Imagine for yourself the impacts of these additional stress factors:

- Activities that push your dog's ability, fitness, or conformation to the limits. This is not all bad, as appropriate challenges are what make us stronger, but pushing limits does carry the risk of excess stress and injury.

- Long toenails that change the angles of the bones in the paws and legs.

- Emotional stresses that impact the body in many ways: affecting breathing, immune system, nervous system, muscle tension, and so on.

- Allergies, excessive flea bites, or hot spots that create inflammation followed by adhesions (gluing) between the skin and underlying tissues.

This list is not complete, but you get the idea. Massage can help recovery from or management of these various stresses by stimulating circulation, easing and balancing muscle tensions, calming nerves—just to name a few examples. The results you can expect will vary depending on many factors, but typically owners who use massage for their dogs are thrilled with the outcome. Am I saying that massage is a magic cure? Of course not—though it can sometimes seem, and even be, miraculous. More often it's the smaller miracles, the ones that may even go unnoticed at first, that add up over time, such as breathing a little more deeply, a more even flow of movement through the hips and tail, climbing stairs more easily, or an increasing inclination to play with toys.

Massage Is Complementary to Chiropractic Care

Another great benefit of massage is helping chiropractic adjustments hold better, hold longer, and even happen more easily in the first place. Dogs may need chiropractic care for all the same reasons they need massage. In fact, it can often be an imbalance of muscle tensions over time that creates chiropractic subluxations ("stuckness" of joints impacting surrounding nerves and tissues). Other causes include rough play, pulls on leashes, accidents, and positions held during surgeries, among many possibilities. It is beyond the scope of this book to cover tips on working with a chiropractor, but it is an important and very related topic, so please visit *www.AllAboutAnimalMassage.com* for more information. For now I can only say please choose your dog's chiropractor with special care and attention, since chiropractic adjustments include greater risk of harm than massage if performed by someone who is not skilled and knowledgeable about both chiropractic care and dog anatomy and health.

For situations when massage is not appropriate (contraindications) see chapter 6: "Guidelines for Effectiveness and Safety," and the website *www.AllAboutAnimalMassage.com*.

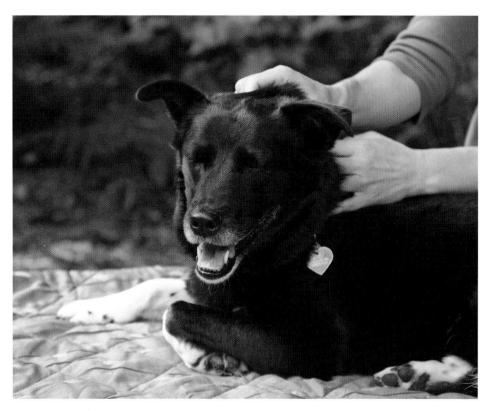

Understanding what is happening for your dog's body will help you apply techniques more effectively.

3
How Massage Works

In chapter 2 we considered a number of stress factors that can affect your dog. Could you see how each of them might have a profound effect on your dog's body? Now read on, and see how the following six concepts can add to what you already know.

Freeing Restrictions: Muscles and Other Soft Tissues

Concept 1: "Glue"—or Restrictions, Adhesions, Knots, and Trigger Points

Two things that happen throughout all bodies at different times, a little here, a lot there, are inflammation and dehydration. Inflammation could be as obvious as a swollen injury, or more invisible like sore, achy muscles after a workout. Dehydration could be for the whole system due to not drinking enough water, but even more often it will involve a smaller area of tissue that's simply not getting a good supply and exchange of fluids, including water, because of tensions, scar tissue, or other restrictions. Inflammation and dehydration both cause the surrounding muscle and other tissues to become less slippery and more sticky. Not only that, but once they start to get sticky, they're also more prone to *(drum roll)* dehydration and inflammation!

As adhesions and restrictions develop, muscles shorten, become even more dehydrated and acidic, develop trigger points and stress points, and generally become dysfunctional. This means they get tired more easily, if they even function properly in the first place. Muscle fatigue and tension, in turn, put extra strain on the tendons and ligaments. Restrictions also create more stress for other structures both near and far, as they work harder trying to compensate and rebalance the body. These other structures may manage to compensate well for a long time, even a lifetime. However, there will always be a price paid at some level eventually, whether as injury, pain, lower energy, less coordination, loss of flexibility, lower endurance, and so on. The good news is that massage is excellent at rehydrating, unsticking, and reducing pain in restrictions such as adhesions and trigger points, whether or not they've yet resulted in a palpable knot.

Relieving Stress: Neurological Effects

Concept 2: Fight or Flight versus Rest and Relaxation

Ever heard of something called stress? Quite the buzz word these days, and for very good reason. It is well worth paying attention to, but without stressing about it, of course! First, take a deep breath. Relax. The good news is that our bodies are well designed to handle stress. In fact, too little stress can be just as much of a problem as too much, since healthy stress stimulates our bodies to becomes stronger, but only if relaxation and recovery are also part of the picture.

Our central nervous system (brain and spinal cord) coordinates activities and sensations throughout our body. Much of this happens without our even thinking about it, such as the regulation of heart rate and blood pressure. Since there are times we need these rates to be high and other times when we don't, the automatic part of our nervous system has two modes that correspond to our different needs: fight or flight and rest and relaxation. The technical terms for these are the *sympathetic* (fight or flight) and the *parasympathetic* (rest and relaxation) systems.

Sympathetic mode is about survival in the short term. In its extreme, it is about saving ourselves from the saber-toothed tiger (or fireworks, lightning storms, fill-in-the-blank) right now. In the less extreme version, it is about anticipating and avoiding the scary or worrisome things in life. Chronic stress means being constantly in this low to moderate state of alarm or worry. Like a broken record, we get in a certain groove and our bodies literally get stuck there, forgetting how to get back into relaxation mode even when we do take a break. This can be as true for animals as it is for us, particularly if we are in this pattern, as they take so many of their cues from the humans in their lives.

Our bodies are designed to work with a *balance* of the two systems. The sympathetic mode is highly useful when we need a burst of strength or activity, but having our bodies revved up all the time would (and often does) wear them out faster than necessary. If we haven't had a chance to really rest, relax, and recover, there will be less energy available for those moments when we really need it.

Great news! Positive touch stimulates the parasympathetic *(para-sym-pa-thet-ic)* nervous system, the rest and relaxation mode. When do you think your body would choose to work on a healing process—while the tiger is chasing you or while you're relaxing? Yes, the physiological processes (in other words, activities of the cells, organs, glands, etc.) that promote healing are stimulated in the parasympathetic state. Examples of the rest and relaxation mode include the following: the heart rate slows; blood vessels dilate (enlarge), which allows better distribution of nutrients; the breath deepens, bringing more oxygen to the blood; waste products and toxins are removed more efficiently; and endorphins (natural painkillers) are produced. If there is tissue damage anywhere, it can get cleaned up and repaired that much quicker. The immune function is better prepared to do its job and fight any enemy cells such as viruses, bacteria, and cancer.

Moving Fluids: Circulatory Effects

Concept 3: Fluid Balance

Every living cell in the body (and that's a really big number, even if you're a Chihuahua) needs fuel delivered to it and waste products taken away, more or less constantly. This delivery system is an important aspect of the body's metabolism, the ability of cells to process nutrients and waste products properly. Without this, the cells can't function properly. Transportation of nutrients and waste products is provided by fluids, but for now let's imagine using delivery trucks and garbage trucks. We'll focus here on the circulation of blood, but there are other fluids in the body, too, such as lymphatic fluid, which we'll look at when we consider the immune system, and also the fluid matrix in and between every cell in the body. We are, after all, about 60 percent water.

How does massage stimulate fluid circulation? And how does that help the body? One way was just mentioned in discussing stress and neurological effects. Remember that part of the relaxation response in the nervous system is to dilate blood vessels. This makes it easier for blood to move along its path. However, there may still be certain areas that have reduced or slowed blood flow due to restrictions, tight muscles, shallow breathing, scar tissue, adhesions, or inflammation. These areas could be as small as the tip of your little finger, as large as the whole body, or anywhere in between. Massage can dramatically improve the thoroughness and efficiency of circulation in these areas by relaxing muscles and mechanically unsticking adhesions and other restrictions. Many massage strokes also directly help move the fluids along their pathways, just like you can "massage" your toothpaste up and out of the top of the tube. (Well, at least a little bit like that.)

For the body as a whole, and on a daily basis, exercise is actually the best way to stimulate circulation. But exercise doesn't always happen for many reasons: injuries, confinement, boredom, arthritis, desk jobs (oops, we're supposed to be focusing on animals). And if we're talking about a specific tight or restricted area, then even exercise won't be enough to get those cells well taken care of. Massage, on the other hand, can be an effective and efficient solution.

> *Staying well hydrated is very important for the health, comfort, and function of all tissues in the body, including muscles.*

Balancing Tensions: Structural Effects

Concept 4: Tensegrity

A big *wow* factor that happens quite often with massage and bodywork is having a pain or tension in one location relieved by a release in a seemingly unconnected body part. In fact, most chronic aches and pains are actually caused by a restriction or imbalance somewhere else in the body, not where the pain is being felt or the movement is being limited. A simplified but also classic example is someone who goes for massage for a sore or tight low back, gets massage in that area, goes home feeling better, and wakes up the next morning with the same low back problem. In this example, it's not until she gets some release for the tight hamstrings (backs of the thighs) that she finally starts making some real progress for her back. Fortunately, there are common patterns that bodyworkers become familiar with, which can help them get more lasting results for their clients more efficiently. These are only general patterns, however. Each individual is unique and there are no cookie-cutter recipes that work for everyone.

The concept that explains how the above wow factor works is known as *tensegrity*. Imagine trying to build a house with only rubber bands. (Okay, let's say it's a very small house.) It would never hold a shape would it? Too flexible, and with no integrity or strength. If you build a house with only strong, rigid parts, though, it may hold its shape nicely for a while, but what if something heavy falls on it or it gets shaken up in an earthquake? It will break because it has no flexibility, no resilience. A tensegrity structure, on the other hand, has a combination of elastic parts (providing tension) and rigid parts (providing integrity) that holds its original shape with a perfect balance of tensions. If something smashes this type of structure down, rather than breaking it simply gets a distorted shape as the tensions are redistributed. When the pressure is released, it pops back to its original shape.

Let's compare this idea to a living body. Many of us likely grew up (so far) thinking that our bones support the rest of our body like bricks in a brick building, one stacked on top of the other, supporting the next one above it, and so on. *Wrong!* Our bodies are tensegrity systems. Our bones are the rigid spacers and our system of muscles and connective tissue, or *fascia*, provides the elastic tension. This is an important distinction when comparing the results of being stressed. If a brick building has one corner smashed that corner is pretty much toast, while the rest of the building may be totally unaffected. This is not how our bodies work. If one part of the body is injured, the whole body is going to experience some effect, whether we notice it or not. The good news, though, is that the whole body can also experience *positive* effect when one part is rebalanced, just as the whole tensegrity structure regains its shape and rebalances tensions when the pressure that was distorting it is released.

When bodywork focuses on this tensegrity quality of our bodies, you can get significant and lasting changes in the alignment of the whole musculo-skeletal system (all the muscles and bones). This results in more efficient posture and movement, which in turn reduces stress, tension, and damage to muscles, joints, and everything else. And by the way, it's not only muscles and bones that are physically linked in this tensegrity system, but also organs, nerves, membranes, blood vessels, the brain, everything! When you hear bodyworkers using terms like fascial work, Structural Integration, Myofascial Release (MFR), or Craniosacral Therapy, among others, they are focusing, at least in part, on skeletal alignment through this tensegrity concept.

By the way, *fascia* with an *sc* is pronounced *fa-shuh* (like *fa-scinating*), or *fah-shuh*, but not *fay-shuh*, which would be spelled *facia*, a different word. You can go to a spa and get a facial, but that's not about fascia!

Efficient Movement: Habits and Patterns

Concept 5: Proprioception *(pro-prio-cep-tion)*

We and our animals all have habitual ways we stand, sit, and move our bodies. Some of these patterns may be efficient and highly functional, but for most of us, including our animals, they are not all so optimal. Good quality physical training that develops strength, flexibility, and balance can improve these habits and patterns dramatically. There are also many forms and aspects of bodywork that focus on the issue of body awareness and movement re-education. Animals, even more so than people, depend on such help from a bodyworker, therapist, or trainer to improve their posture and dysfunctional patterns of movement.

How do changes in movement patterns occur, for better or worse? Proprioception. There are specialized cells throughout the body called proprioceptors, primarily in and around joints. These cells send signals to the brain about position in and movement through space. Proprioception is the key difference between a talented, agile athlete and a well-conditioned klutz. The better the proprioception, the better the communication between the brain and the body. But when the brain learns, whether by habit or as a response to injury, that the movement available at a joint is less than perfect, it will continue to move only within that range until any problem (swelling, pain, adhesion, etc.) is resolved, and also until the proprioceptors and the brain are retrained to recognize the full potential again, the full range of motion.

A classic example is someone walking with a limp even after a broken bone has healed and the cast has been removed. But poor or dysfunctional proprioception can also happen without injury, simply by lack of movement or due to emotional patterns expressed in posture, for example. If the body doesn't use each joint in all ranges of motion for which it was designed, at least once in a while, then over time the system will forget what was actually the true normal, the full potential, and settle for whatever is used in the habitual movements. Quality training, bodywork, and stretching can all effectively give positive input to the proprioceptor cells in and around the joints, improving proprioception and efficiency of movement and posture.

Promoting Health: Immune Function

Concept 6: The Lymphatic System

How does the immune system work to protect the body against disease, and how does massage support it? All physical systems of our bodies (circulatory, lymphatic, neurological, digestive, respiratory, etc.) actually contribute to immune function. Elements such as physical barriers (skin and connective tissue), good bacteria (on the skin and in the digestive system), pH balancing, temperature regulation, special cells that fight germs, transportation of fighter cells and waste products through lymph vessels, lymph nodes that filter and cleanse the lymph fluid—all of these and more play a part in the body's ability to resist and recover from illness.

What role does massage play? For one thing, look back at concept 2. The immune system is supported and stimulated when the rest and relaxation mode is dominant. Circulation (concept 3) is another key; for the blood, yes, but also for the circulation of the lymphatic system, which is what we'll focus on now. This system operates much like the system of veins for blood, including the fact that exercise and massage are two of the best ways to stimulate it. The main difference is that rather than transporting blood cells and plasma, it's transporting lymph fluid. Lymph, like the blood, acts as both delivery trucks and garbage trucks for all cells in the body. But the deliveries are more focused on situations needing repair (injuries and infections), and the garbage trucks are focused on slightly different items, maybe we could say more of the actual garbage versus the recycling bins.

Virtually any massage will have positive effects for the immune system, though it is also possible to experience (temporarily) some flu-like symptoms following a massage. This is usually because there have been lots of waste products piling up (garbage trucks on strike?). When you draw the body's attention to it and finally tackle the now much bigger job, it is bound to be uncomfortable for a while. Would you rather continue in denial and let the garbage keep piling up? I hope not!

Lymphatic massage (also known as Lymphatic Facilitation or Manual Lymphatic Drainage) focuses on moving fluids along this delicate lymphatic system. It is often used with great success to reduce edema (swelling), but it also supports the general immune function of the body.

These six concepts should give you plenty to think about, for your animals and for yourself. There is just so much going on in the body, and so many ways that massage can support it: in muscle comfort, strength, and flexibility; in relaxation and reduced stress; in circulation and metabolism; in efficient alignment, posture, and movement; and in healthy immune function. I encourage you to return to this chapter and read about the concepts again, one at a time, as you massage your dog using the techniques you will learn in chapter 7. Remember, too, that you can find many resources to deepen your understanding of these physiological processes and anatomy, as well as other massage topics, by going to *www.AllAboutAnimalMassage.com* and asking questions, reading articles, newsletters, and books, and interacting with others through the "Animal Wellness Network."

4
Adaptation Versus Healing

After having read the previous chapters, it may seem miraculous to you that any of our animals, or us for that matter, have ever survived without regular massage. While this is an admirable feat (you can ask any massage therapist), the evidence suggests that it is indeed possible, and there are two main reasons for this. One is movement. Move it or lose it, so they say. (Fortunately, exercise is hugely beneficial to our health. Unfortunately, we don't tend to move quite as much as our ancestors did, nor do most of our animals.) Another reason is that so often our survival is managed more by *adaptation* to an injury or other problem than by fully healing from it.

Fortunately, Unfortunately

In fact, the process of recovery from an injury all too often can be described as a continuous cycle of "fortunately, unfortunately, fortunately, unfortunately . . ."

- Fortunately, our bodies have amazing powers to adapt and change as needed.
- Unfortunately, this process of adaptation can often create new challenges.

Picture a mildly traumatic injury, such as a dog being barreled over by a larger playmate. Say there is some bruising, and various ligaments and tissues are strained in the effort first to avoid and then to recover from falling.

- Fortunately, the body sends various elements (delivered in blood and lymph) to clean up damaged tissue and make repairs.
- Unfortunately, these elements arrive in excess fluid (edema, or swelling), which increases pressure and pain in the area.
- Fortunately, this pain can help remind the body to move carefully while repairs are underway.
- Unfortunately, some of the fluid tends to hang around much longer than it needs to, partly due to the lack of movement already mentioned. It then becomes thicker and stickier, i.e. gluey, and adhesions and restrictions begin to develop.

- Fortunately, there now seems to be less suffering because the body is adapting to the restricted movement and pain, learning to recognize a new "normal" as proprioception adapts to the new situation.

- Unfortunately, now various structures (muscle, bone, tendon, ligaments, blood vessels, nerves, you name it) are, in fact, glued together (adhesions) and range of motion (movement) is physically restricted.

- Fortunately, the body has many other parts, near and far, which can make up for this compromised and restricted area's shortcomings. This is known as compensation.

- Unfortunately, this eventually leads to the same cycle of stress and strain for those parts doing the compensating, because they are now having to work overtime.

This scenario works much the same for repetitive stress type injuries as it does for more traumatic ones, like the fall in this example. Of course, the power of our bodies to adapt in these ways really *is* quite amazing and highly useful, just also less than perfect. *Fortunately*, what the body can do, it can generally undo, with a little help. Interventions like massage and other therapies can transform the scenario above to one where restrictions are released or even prevented in the first place, full range of motion is restored, and compensation patterns are no longer needed as the whole system returns to its original balance.

Injuries: A Team Approach

An injured animal will ideally have a team of care providers. You, your veterinarian, the trainer if you have one, and your massage professional are key members of the team. Massage can be a practical and compassionate way to help your dog when she has been injured. It's important to remember that during recovery from an injury, surgery, or other trauma, an animal's massage needs are going to be different from the normal routine. An injured animal's veterinarian should be consulted and give consent before beginning a program of therapeutic massage.

In the early stages of healing, specific techniques such as Manual Lymphatic Drainage can help decrease swelling and support the immune system. Further into the healing process, scar tissue can be effectively worked with to prevent adhesions and promote functional arrangement of the fibers, helping the scar tissue itself develop with optimal strength and flexibility. And further along still, appropriate stretches and other techniques can help range of motion and body awareness return more completely and positively.

Throughout the entire recovery period, massage can also be used to support the rest of the body, working to alleviate patterns of stress and compensation, including those patterns that may have contributed to the injury in the first place. Massage can be very helpful to relieve boredom and depression during recovery from an injury or illness. Heightened feelings of well-being greatly enhance the healing process.

When an animal is recovering from an injury, the advanced training and expertise of a massage professional can support her in many ways. The therapist will want to see the animal at certain intervals, which will vary depending on the trauma, the other treatments received (including those you provide), the goals for recovery, and resources (time, finances, experience, etc.).

In between the professional sessions, there is much that you can do to support the healing process and the work begun by the bodyworker. During rehabilitation, daily attention, even multiple times a day, can be extremely helpful. Be sure to use the professional as a teacher to show you what's most appropriate and beneficial for your dog's needs. He can make decisions about prioritizing goals; about which techniques to use, when, and how often; about which directions to work, how much pressure to use, and so on. In any therapeutic situation, you and your massage professional have the same goal—your dog's health and well-being—and he will be happy to work with you and your veterinarian in a team approach.

The body is a healing machine. It wants to be balanced and is capable of rebalancing itself (potentially, if also imperfectly). Any modality that helps the body be more connected within itself, and on multiple levels, will help it function closer and closer to its potential.

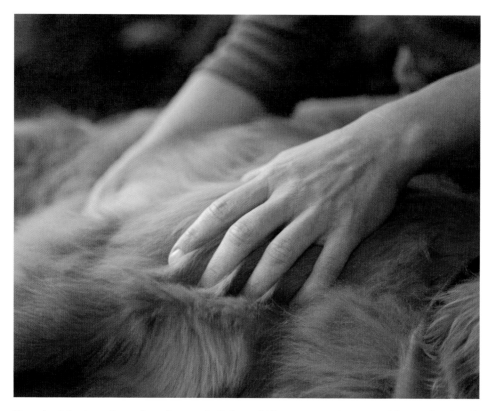

Your dog's body and your learning can both benefit from an appointment with a professional.

5
Finding and Working with a Massage Professional

Part two of this book will give you many massage techniques you can use for your dog. Let's say you've been massaging your dog on your own. When and why would you decide to call in a professional? Here are some scenarios where a professional bodyworker or massage therapist can help you and your dog.

- You're noticing a pattern of tension, pain, or restricted range of motion with which you'd like to make better progress.

- You'd like a professional's assessment of your dog's tension patterns that your level of skill and experience may not detect.

- Your dog sustains an injury and needs the more advanced skills of a professional.

- You and your dog have a competition or other event coming up, and you want your dog to have every possible advantage.

- You want to observe and learn more from what a professional bodyworker can show you in person.

- You love the idea of regular massage for your dog, but just don't have time to do it yourself.

It is very important to understand that massage and bodywork professionals are neither trained nor licensed to provide any diagnosis, prognosis, or medical treatment of any kind. Always call your veterinarian first if there is even a suspicion that there is a current medical situation such as an injury or illness. If your veterinarian approves, the therapist can provide appropriate, supportive complementary attention, such as massaging areas of the body that are working to compensate for an injury, or promoting relaxation, circulation, healing, and many other benefits.

How do you go about finding a professional and scheduling an appointment? What should you ask? What should you expect from her, and what might she expect from you? Does your state regulate animal massage, and if so, what qualifications are required?

To find a massage therapist or bodyworker for your dog, start by asking other professionals such as your trainer, veterinarian, or groomer if they have recommendations. If you take your dog to a kennel or doggie daycare, they may also provide massage or be able to give you referrals. Of course, another excellent approach is asking friends and acquaintances who they've worked with and if they've experienced positive results. You can expand your list of options further with resources on the Internet, including my website, *www. AllAboutAnimalMassage.com*, where you can do a search within our "Animal Wellness Network" for animal care professionals near you, including massage therapists and bodyworkers. Pet stores often have bulletin boards with business cards and fliers from local professionals, as well. And of course, you can find advertisements in dog-related publications and at events like shows and expos.

You and Your Professional: Working Together

Before, during, and after your appointment, there are specific things you can ask and do to optimize the experience for you and your dog, and to assist the professional in doing the best job for you. Your observation skills during the first appointment, the following days, and over the next few appointments will help you learn more about the therapist's work and your dog's body and responses.

Questions to ask before making an appointment

Q: *Can you tell me about your experience, training, certification, licensing, background, specialty, approach, etc? (Choose one or two or more words that work for you. You can also ask for references from among her clients.)*

A: Many answers could be fine, depending on your animal's needs, your goals, and any regulations existing in the state you live in (see "Regulations," page 30). As a point of reference, most certification programs for animal massage are between 50 and several hundred hours. Most licensing or certification programs for human massage are 500 to 1000 hours. You can get some sense of where the therapist falls within these ranges, though remember that continuing education hours (training taken after initial certification or licensing) are also significant. Of course, experience is also important but typically harder to measure or compare, so just listen and get your own sense as best you can.

Q: *What are your rates?*

A: A useful comparison is the rates in your area for massage or bodywork for people. Although that's generally going to cover a wide range, you can get a sense of the average and expect a similar range for animal massage. However, if you drive your dog to the therapist, and since dog massages are typically under an hour, the rates may be a bit less than for a one-hour human massage.

Q: *Do I need to be there for the appointment? (Assuming it will be someplace other than your home, like a boarding facility, doggie daycare, groomer, or your veterinarian's office.)*

A: Of course it's best that someone who knows your dog be there at least for the first appointment. Some therapists may require the owner to be present at the first or all appointments, which could relate to their philosophy, modality (type of bodywork), dog-handling skills, past experiences, or any combination of these or other factors. Many professionals are willing to work without the owner there once they know the dog, which is an obvious benefit to scheduling ease.

Q: *Do you prefer to work before or after my dog gets exercised, fed, etc?*

A: This may be partly dependent on the information you provide about your dog's routines, energy level, issues, distractions, and what the goals are for the session. It is ideal to find a time of day that the distractions will be minimal, so your dog can best focus on and receive the bodywork.

Q: *If another event is also on your dog's calendar, such as a show, long hike, chiropractic appointment, acupuncture, or other veterinary appointment: Is it best to schedule the bodywork for before or after the appointment or event? How soon before or after?*

A: You may need to coordinate some communication between the massage professional and veterinarian, or anyone else involved. What are the goals for the bodywork session? Is it to prepare your dog for an upcoming event or help him to recover from it, or both? Has the dog received bodywork before? If he has, his responses will be more predictable than if he hasn't. This may affect decisions about timing, since the changes produced by massage may take the dog a day or two to adjust to. Regarding chiropractic care, my experience is that massage either before or after can be just fine, with different advantages to each. Whichever work comes first, the next professional's work is supported by the progress already made. If the dog is lame or in apparent pain, you should first call the veterinarian, who may also be the chiropractor. In each individual case, it will be best simply to ask any professionals involved, beginning with your veterinarian, about what their preferences and advice are.

Q: *What is your cancellation policy?*

A: Many will have one, some may not. The more notice you can give, the more helpful it is. Of course, it's also helpful for each of you to have a phone number to call for updates and last minute changes.

Being prepared for the appointment

- Have your dog clean and dry.

- Allow your therapist some flexibility in timing, or make it clear when scheduling if you can't. Though you should expect her to respect your time, driving from place to place can make timing a challenge for the therapist.

- Be ready to give information relating to your dog's behavior, medical conditions, medications, past injuries, surgeries, etc.

During the appointment

- A great thing to do during the session is to focus on your own breathing. This will help your dog and will also help you stay tuned in to his responses and communication.

- Avoid petting, grooming, feeding, or excessive or loud talking during the massage. This can be distracting and potentially interfere with your dog's focus, his communication with the therapist, and the results achieved. Of course sometimes your touch, handling, or voice may be helpful, so ask the therapist what she prefers.

- Watch what the therapist does and ask questions about things you can do yourself between sessions.

- Observe how often your dog seems tuned into his own body and how much he seems to participate in the process with the therapist versus either ignoring or resisting the work. Keep in mind that distractions in the environment can interfere with this, for some dogs more than others. There is also a definite learning process to receiving bodywork. For some dogs it takes about a minute to figure it out. For others it can take several sessions or more. For most it's somewhere in between.

- Signs of relaxation and release during the session (lying down, soft eyes, yawning, deeper breathing, etc.) are positive. Even more important are the effects you'll notice over the next several days. Also look at cumulative changes over the course of several sessions.

- Don't judge the session by whether your dog falls asleep or is doing advanced yoga by the end, nor by whether the therapist looks like she's working hard, talks with a lot of technical terms, or charges a lot of money.

- Expect some ebb and flow between states of focus, relaxation, and even temporary agitation when an area is sore or compromised in some way. Does the therapist help your dog through these challenges in a positive manner? Is the area left alone because the dog doesn't like it? This option may be a great temporary solution for the sake of trust building or to get some releases happening elsewhere in the body, but an area of concern needs to be addressed, or actively worked toward, unless it's beyond the skill or scope of the therapist.

At the end of the appointment

- Expect the professional to tell you her observations about your dog's areas of tension, indications of restrictions, tenderness, pain, or worry. She will also often tell you whether range of motion for various joints was normal or reduced, or triggered a pain response. She may watch your dog move and share observations about that and about general posture. Additional, specific observations and language may vary depending on the therapist and the type of bodywork being done.

- You should not expect or ask for a diagnosis of any kind. Nor can the therapist tell you specifically why your dog has certain tensions, restrictions, or discomforts. She *can*, however, teach you about how the body works and why certain types of causes can lead to certain types of effects.

- Each dog is completely individual and so will be the healing process. For this reason, the professional won't be able to tell you how long improvements will take or even whether massage will produce your desired results. She may be able to share some examples of what has happened for other clients in similar situations, though, which can give you a sense of what is possible.

After the massage

- Be sure your dog has water available, and also a chance to relieve himself. The changes that happen during bodywork often require a more than usual amount of the body's water for processing, resulting in thirst and a full bladder.

- If possible, give your dog a chance to move around soon after the session to integrate the changes that happened during the massage. This helps his awareness and proprioception integrate the releases of restrictions, increases in range of motion, and increases in comfort.

- Using your own judgment, follow the bodyworker's recommendations about exercise, rest, or appointments. You are ultimately responsible for choosing which advice to follow for the sake of your dog and for yourself. If you choose not to follow the recommendations, however, you may or may not get the results you're looking for, or as quickly as you might hope.

- Observe your dog over the next few days and weeks. Does his movement, mood, or energy level change? How does he behave? How does he respond when you groom him? Does he hold his tail or head and neck differently? Have a change in appetite?

- Do feel free to call and talk with the professional as needed between sessions, whether to ask questions about your observations or about the follow-up recommendations she may have made. She will also generally welcome hearing about your observations since the previous session.

- Does your dog have any stiffness the first day or two after the session? Stiffness can mean several different things. It could be due to excessive pressures or techniques used by the therapist, but it could just as easily be due to the natural healing process, release of toxins, rebalancing tensions, strengthening weaker muscles, and so forth. If you have any concerns about your dog's responses, be sure to call the therapist and/or your dog's veterinarian to discuss your observations.

- Give the therapist feedback, either at the next appointment or sooner, about your observations. Remember, you are a team.

Scheduling the next appointment

- Recommendations from the professional for the timing of the next session will vary depending on how your dog is doing, what the goals are, and in some cases the type of bodywork being done.

- For new clients, I find it helpful to schedule a second session fairly soon, say within one to three weeks, if there are some significant issues to be addressed. A longer interval is fine if the dog seems to be doing quite well. Of course, more often is always beneficial for prevention and maintenance, if you prefer that for your dog.

- By the end of the second session you will have much more information, including your observations during the interim since the first appointment. This will give you a better idea of how quickly your dog is responding to massage.

- Looking at your goals together, you and the therapist can both then better estimate the optimal frequency of sessions going forward. As time goes on, adjustments to the plan can be made as the situation develops.

Creating a working relationship with a professional bodyworker may take a little time. Use your own judgment, observation, and intuition when deciding whether to continue making appointments with the same person, try someone new, or do a combination of both. You may want to try more than one appointment before making a decision, though. Your dog may need some time to develop trust. There may be significant pain or imbalance issues that simply take more time to address. Remember that progress is not always obvious or measurable, and it's natural that some sessions will produce more obvious results than others. Countless factors contribute to the fact that each session is different. If you don't feel a clear sense of benefit after a few sessions, however, I would encourage you to consider another person.

Take Care of Yourself for Your Dog's Sake

Your own personal familiarity with massage and other forms of bodywork can benefit your dog. The more you receive bodywork yourself, the more educated you will become as a receiver and consumer. This in turn will help you in making decisions about services for your animals. It's remarkable how often body issues and tension patterns are mirrored between animal and owner, and addressing both together can provide even more progress than supporting only one of the partners.

Some therapists are licensed to work on both people and animals. In this case, you and your dog may have the opportunity to receive bodywork from the same person, which can give you very direct information about his work. Don't rule out the therapist who does not do people, however. Many excellent therapists prefer to devote themselves to helping our animal companions.

What's In a Name?

In most cases, the term a professional uses to describe himself will tell you very little about his qualifications. Here are just a few samples of labels you may come across, but know that you will still want to be asking questions about training and experience.

When it comes to animal massage, any of the labels listed below generally will be prefaced with Horse/Equine, Dog/Canine, Large Animal/Small Animal, Cat/Feline, etc. The title may also begin with Licensed or Certified. Licensed means that your state has some official means of licensing individuals for the profession, and that this individual has been through that process. Certified means he's taken a course that gave him a certificate at the end, but it doesn't tell you about what that course involved.

You will come across titles like Massage Therapist, Massage Practitioner, Bodyworker, Sports Massage Therapist, Acupressure or Shiatsu Practitioner, Structural Integration Practitioner, Rolfer, etc. More terms exist, but these are some of the more common. Some terms are specifically trademarked by a particular school and can only be used by those graduates.

Interestingly, I've come across some objection to using the terms *therapist* or *practitioner* at all in referring to animal massage, even though these are the terms most often used by massage professionals for people. One suggestion (not my own) is that we use the term Massage Provider instead, also a perfectly useful title. Such distinction in terms is closely intertwined with the whole issue of whether animal massage constitutes practicing veterinary medicine, an on-going hot topic in many states.

Regulations

What follows is some much-abbreviated information on regulations related to animal massage, for your education and interest. You do not need to feel responsible for this information in seeking services for your animals. It is the provider's responsibility to understand any regulations applying to the work in his own state if he's in business and charging for services.

The legal question of animal massage is a still-evolving issue that varies from state to state, year to year, day to day, and also sometimes according to your information source. Many states do have regulations, and many more are in the process of determining them. Some states include massage in the definition of "veterinary medicine," and therefore do not allow it outside of veterinary practices. There is great debate about whether this approach or any other form of regulation is an appropriate solution. You may choose to ignore the issue, or gather information from people you know, including your veterinarian. Or you may feel inclined to research it thoroughly online. You may even feel inclined to become involved with your own state's decisions about this aspect of animal care.

One resource that you may find helpful is the International Association of Animal Massage and Bodywork. You can find this association online via a link on *www.AllAboutAnimalMassage.com,* or through an Internet search engine. The IAAMB is a professional organization for animal massage therapists and bodyworkers, though membership is open to anyone who supports animal massage. Their website includes information on laws and regulations by state. The IAAMB chart on the topic is very handy and informative, though they can't be held responsible for guaranteeing that the information is always completely up-to-date. They do have updates on news from various states as issues come up. They also provide links and guidance to go directly to your own state's legislative website to research the current situation in your state.

> *Why, you may ask, doesn't this book include pictures and names of all the muscles? Well, at a beginning stage it really won't help you learn massage. The anatomy included with each technique in part two will give you a great start, however. When and if you are interested in learning more anatomy, please visit* www.AllAboutAnimalMassage.com *for resources.*

Part Two

Massaging Your Dog

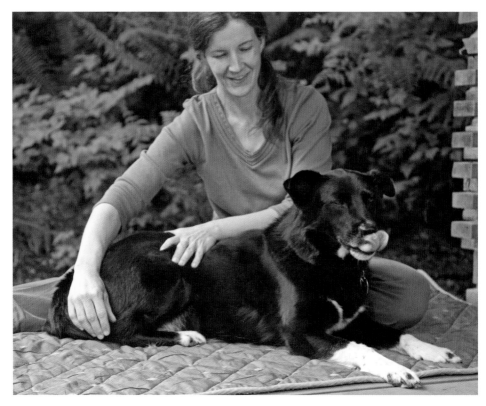

An effective and safe position for massaging your dog is comfortable for you, secure for your dog, and does not put your face too close to your dog's.

6

Guidelines for
Effectiveness and Safety

> *Before you begin massaging your dog, know that massage is not a substitute for proper veterinary care. Please do not delay in calling your veterinarian if your dog is in pain or showing any symptoms of injury or illness.*

Contraindications and Precautions

For healthy animals, there is little worry about causing any harm with massage as long as you are using reasonable judgment about the pressures you use and always pay attention to your dog's feedback. If your dog has an illness, injury, or medical condition, certain types of massage and bodywork can still be very beneficial to aid the healing process. However, in these cases the effects of massage could also be harmful, depending on the specific condition, whether the symptoms are acute, and what techniques are used and how they are applied. Before massaging any animal with an illness, injury, or medical condition, be sure to consult with your veterinarian.

- Do not massage any animal who has a fever or systemic infection, or one who is in a state of shock.

- Do not massage directly over areas of current injury, local infection, skin condition, or recent surgery.

- If you have any question about whether certain techniques or massage in general are appropriate for your animal's medical situation, please ask your veterinarian. This includes, but is not limited to, conditions involving the heart, kidneys, liver, and circulation.

It is possible that your dog could experience adverse reactions during or after a massage. This may depend on underlying conditions, past experiences, remnants of past medications or anesthesia in the body, or massage techniques being applied too intensely for that individual. Typically, any adverse reactions are temporary and a natural part of the healing process as the body releases stagnant waste products, toxins, emotions, and restrictions. Examples include muscle stiffness or a change in energy level. If your dog received a massage from someone other than yourself, you should call that person to discuss your observations. If you have any concerns, or if the reactions persist more than one or two days, consult with your veterinarian.

Although a few safety and handling suggestions are included, the intent of this book is not to teach animal handling. It is assumed that you will be working with your own animal, that you are familiar with your animal, and that you already know how to handle her safely and effectively. If you have questions about this for your situation, please consult a professional to help you.

The techniques I've chosen for chapter 7 are moves I use regularly in my own practice. They will help you monitor, support, and learn about your dog's body as you massage. I find them to be highly effective and easy to teach and learn. However, like many of the simplest arts, their effectiveness and your skill with them can be developed over a lifetime. I invite you and encourage you to return to this book and to the resources you will find at *www.AllAboutAnimalMassage.com* as you continue to learn and practice. Not only will you add new tools to your "toolbox" this way, but you will also continue to refine and rediscover the ones you've already learned. And remember that receiving massage is one of the very best ways to learn about giving massage, with some pretty great additional benefits as a bonus!

Effectiveness

> *"Whether you think you can, or you think you can't, either way, you are right."* —Henry Ford

Steps

1. Know that you *can* massage your dog effectively.

2. Listen to what your dog tells you.

3. Listen to your intuition.

4. Visualize positive results.

5. Keep on learning.

6. Keep on massaging!

Of course, your most important teacher in this lifelong learning process will be your dog through the honest feedback she gives you. Although humans can (but often don't) give detailed, verbal feedback, the nonverbal feedback from the dogs you massage will be constant, accurate, and very helpful, if you pay attention and recognize the responses. Since looking directly into dogs' eyes can make them nervous, use soft, intermittent glances to observe your dog's expression. She will tell you when to speed up, slow down, lighten up, or go deeper. She will tell you where she is tight, whether she's also sore, just a little worried, or especially focused. She may even show you where you should massage next.

As you massage, you will gather information largely from your dog's responses, but also from what your hands detect as they palpate (feel) her body. With practice you will increase your ability to feel evidence of less healthy or restricted tissue with your hands. This sensitivity will continue to develop as long as you continue practicing, even over a lifetime. The areas of tension and restriction may feel a number of different ways depending on just what is going on and for how long. They may feel like dryness: not like the skin is wet or dry but as if you're massaging a dry sponge rather than a slighlty moist sponge, or dry clay versus moist clay. You may also feel that the tissue feels hard, gluey, or sticky, or has an uneven texture. You might notice that two structures (such as skin and underlying muscle, or two neighboring muscles) move as one lump mass rather than having some glide between them. Or you may not notice the sensations in your hands at all, but your dog may show a pain response or simply look at you differently or hold her breath.

Being able to confidently interpret all that your dog is telling you or what you feel with your hands is sometimes another story, however. Below are some tips to get you started. For more information related to these tips and others, I recommend *Massaging My Dog: A Guided Journal*, available as an e-book at *www.AllAboutAnimalMassage.com*. This journal is an interactive workbook containing questions and charts to guide you and help you record your observations. It includes additional information on interpreting your dog's feedback, movement, and posture; on what you feel with your hands and intuition; and on the results of the techniques. Not only will the journal support your development in all of these skills, but you will also end up with a record of the patterns in your dog's body and the changes that occur over time.

Top 10 Tips for Observing Your Dog's Feedback and Patterns

1.   There are many signs of a release happening or the positive effect of your touch. These signs include relaxing muscles or posture, sleepy or soft eyes, licking and chewing, a sigh, deeper breathing, yawning, and releasing gas. (Any release is a good release, so I've heard!)

2.   Signs of discomfort, pain, or ticklishness, or the anticipation of any of these, are all significant and can be improved (decreased) with bodywork. These include moving away, holding the breath, excessive panting, tensing muscles, curled lips, biting (gentle or otherwise), or simply a worried look in the eye.

3. A dog's yawns may be a sign of either release and relaxation or of stress. The two types each have a different feel and look to them, which you can learn to recognize by noticing what other body language and feedback signals your dog is giving you at the same time.

4. Some dogs will give more subtle feedback than others, based on their experiences, training, and personality, as well as on how sore they are. You can also expect, over time, that your dog will learn to give more subtle, polite, and accurate feedback if you are paying attention and responding to it.

5. Compare left and right sides of the body in checking for reactions, heat or coldness, swelling, tension, mobility of joints or tissues, or textures such as the following: dry, gluey, sticky, thickened, hard, spongy, bumpy, squishy, zingy, along with the other descriptions you will create as you find them.

6. Always thank your dog (out loud or silently) when she gives you some feedback. Even negative feedback is helpful information, as long as your safety is not compromised.

7. If your dog gives negative feedback signals (such as listed in number 2, above), you will need to find a balance between respecting her communication and being persistent in order to help her. While there are times to use some restraint for your safety, you must never *inflict* the massage on your dog. It is always possible to find some compromise, in time if not right away. You have many options. You can leave the area for now, knowing you will return to it later. You can persist but with a variation of pressure, speed, or technique. Perhaps all you need to change is your own breathing, and relax. You can also enlist the help of a professional to work with your dog and to coach you.

8. Don't assume that the goal is to put your dog to sleep, though certainly relaxation is a positive sign. It is quite natural for your dog to go through waves of relaxation, alternating with higher energy and a desire to move. How much of each can depend on the application of the massage, but also on your dog's age, energy level, attention span, experience with bodywork, the time of day, and countless distractions and expectations, not to mention the degree of soreness.

9. Each observation you make is just one piece of information. Pay attention to it, remember it, even go ahead and assume it's significant, but also know that it may not mean exactly what it seems at first. The more observations you make that point toward the same conclusion, the more confidently you can make that interpretation.

10. Always pay attention to your intuition. There are more ways to receive information than just observation of body language or through palpation (touch).

Safety

The aspects of safety that apply most directly to this book are restraint and your own body mechanics.

Restraint

If you are massaging your dog on a table (which should only be done with nonslip padding), effective restraint is very important to ensure that she doesn't jump or fall and injure herself. For small dogs or dogs with joint issues, injuries, stitches, etc., even the height of a couch or bed could put them at risk.

Depending on your dog's needs, the location of your session, and your own goals and preferences, a leash can be helpful during a session to allow your dog some freedom of movement and still maintain control.

Body Mechanics

Look for examples of the following guidelines in the photographs in chapter 7.
As much as possible:

1. Keep your back comfortably straight and upright, whether sitting, kneeling, or standing.

2. Sitting on the floor with your dog works well in many cases, but other options may include having your dog sit or lie on your lap, or on a sofa, bed, or table. These choices will depend on his size, your body's comfort, the rules of the house, and safety concerns. (If massaging up on furniture, see the safety information above, under "Restraint.")

3. Keep your wrists, fingers, and thumbs well aligned anytime you are using them to apply pressure. For the wrist and fingers this means straight or slightly flexed, not hyperextended. For the thumb this means in line with your forearm rather than straight out to the side.

4. When you use fingers and/or thumbs, use them together to support each other like splints rather than spread out too much.

5. Keep your shoulders relaxed and down.

6. Breathe! This will help your body in every way, including oxygen supply and keeping your joints and muscles from stiffening.

Therapeutic Petting and Grooming

Try these three simple steps to add a therapeutic element to your everyday petting and grooming routines, as well as whenever you practice massage. By using the special techniques of breathing, listening, and visualizing, you will enhance communication with your dog and increase your ability to use therapeutic touch.

1. **Breathe.** It is amazing how powerfully therapeutic something as simple as the breath can be. Use your breath both to connect more completely with your dog and also to encourage him to breathe more regularly and deeply. People and animals alike hold the breath for any number of reasons: pain, worry, fear, stress, and also simply out of habit. When we shift to regular, deep, easy breathing (in and out the nose as much as possible), it relaxes and balances our nervous system and the health of our tissues.

    It is easy to forget and start holding your breath again when you are concentrating on something, like massaging your dog, for example. So give yourself frequent reminders. You might even make a sign or other visual reminder for yourself. You can also time your breath with the hand or brush strokes. This works quite beautifully. The more you practice, the more naturally the breath will flow, enhancing any massage you do. And you will benefit as much from the process as your dog.

    A great exercise for learning to breathe while you massage is to try the opposite, purposely hold your breath while massaging. (Well, just hold some breaths, and the rest of the time shallow breathing. You still need to stay conscious!) This way you can directly experience just how much better it feels, and how much better your dog will respond, when you do *breathe*!

2. **Listen.** In this special kind of listening you will primarily be using your hands, eyes, intuition, and heart. You can, of course, also use your ears to include any sounds your dog makes. Constantly observe, and let your dog know that you are observing by responding to his feedback. Does he turn to look at you or a part of his body? Does he hold his breath? Does he move into or away from something? Notice if his eye is soft (relaxed, happy) or hard (worried, tense).

    A massage is not something you do to your dog, but rather a constant conversation between his body and your hands. If you expect him to participate with you, you must always be listening to his part of the conversation. The more you practice together, the more your dog will tell you about what's going on in his body and mind.

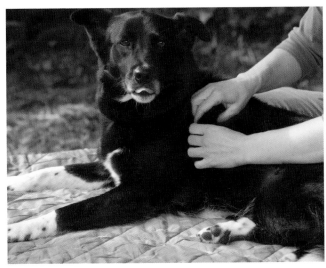

Listen when your dog shows any tension or worry, and respond with a change, such as lightening up, slowing down, or changing the type of stroke.

Then notice when a positive change occurs, such as the softer eyes and more relaxed posture in this photo.

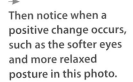

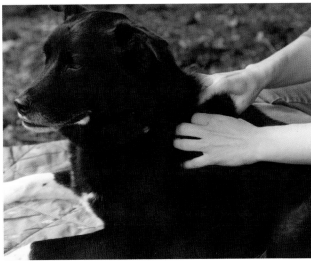

3. **Visualize.** Picture the goal. Focus on what you want, rather than what you don't want. If your dog is holding his breath, for example, or showing tension in some other way, keep visualizing his breath deepening and his body relaxing, rather than focusing on the tension. You can also visualize what's happening under the skin, such as blood flow increasing, adhesions melting, or nerves calming. Your ability to visualize will deepen with practice. The more you experience the changes you visualize, feeling them under your hands or observing them in your dog's body language, the more clearly and vividly you can picture them happening beforehand, and the more powerful your visualizations become.

Top Three Resources for Learning More Massage Skills

1. The ultimate resource, your dog! He or she can teach you (almost) everything you want to know.

2. Visit *www.AllAboutAnimalMassage.com*, where you can find classes and schools, video clips, articles, DVDs, books, tools, professional services, other websites and organizations, the "All About Animal Massage" newsletter, and more. You can also visit and join our "Animal Wellness Network," which connects you with other people around topics of caring for our animals, including massage and bodywork. A treasure trove of information to assist you in your learning adventure.

3. Have a professional massage your dog. Watch what she does; observe your dog's responses. Ask the professional to teach and advise you on your own dog's body.

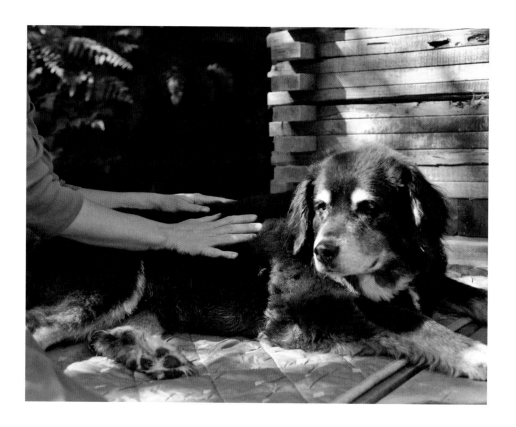

7
Nine Basic Techniques
with Anatomy Connections

General Directions
Building Your Skills and Creating Sessions

Choose one or two new techniques to focus on learning during each session that you share with your dog. This will help keep the experience even more positive for both of you. Each session you do (after the first), begin by reviewing some of the techniques you've already practiced, and then add the new one or two for the day. I've arranged them in a sequence that works well to build on, eventually putting them together to create a basic, full-body massage. You don't have to go in this order, however. By following the guidelines below for creating a session, combined with reading your dog's feedback as discussed in chapter 6, you will learn to tailor each massage to your dog's own needs for that day.

When you're familiar with all nine techniques here, as well as some of the variations suggested, you will find many more techniques to learn from the following resources. *More Massage Moves for Dog Lovers* is an e-book available at *www.AllAboutAnimalMassage.com*. It contains additional Techniques, Anatomy Connections, and Coaching Tips to help you continue to build on all you learn here.

Most of the information in *More Massage Moves* is adapted from *The Horse Lover's Guide to Massage*, so if you are a horse lover, you may choose to purchase the book, adapting the techniques to your dog yourself.

You can also find more to learn in the free "All About Animal Massage" newsletter, and the articles, books, DVDs, and other resources available at *www.AllAboutAnimalMassage.com*.

Creating a Session

Choose a time of day and a location such that you and your dog can both focus, relax, and enjoy the process. Often a little before bedtime works well, especially if you have a high-energy dog. (Remember that she may need to go outside again before bed to release fluids following a massage.) As her body learns to associate massage and relaxation in this way, you can use massage at other times of the day to help calm her.

It is important that there be some form of a beginning and an end to each session, a touch version of "Hello, would you like a massage?" and "Thank you, time to end now." Full Body Stroking (Technique 1) makes an excellent opening and closing for any massage. There are other options, too, such as a quiet touch on the back, chest, or head, and simply breathing some easy breaths together. Do also always begin by asking your dog's permission and end with a thank you.

When transitioning from one technique to another, or one area of the body to another, use long strokes (as with Full Body Stroking) to connect your work. For example, if you just finished a technique for the neck and next you want to do a shoulder technique, use strokes from where you just had your hands on the neck to connect into the shoulder before starting that next technique. This will be much more pleasing to your dog and will also give her a clearer sensation of how the different areas of her body connect to each other and to her brain and awareness.

Always (when it works) have both hands touching your dog. Sometimes both hands will be active for the technique, but even when one hand is not active, it is still involved and connected for a supportive and grounding effect.

Choose one or two Coaching Tips to particularly focus on as you practice. For example, for Full Body Stroking you might choose using soft hands and visualizing blood flow. You can mix and match Coaching Tips with other techniques in many cases.

Variations: You can also mix and match techniques with different areas of the body. For example, try vibrations over the hip joints, kneading the hamstrings along the back of your dog's thigh, or tapotement on the chest. The more you practice, the more you will use your creativity to discover new combinations.

Length of Sessions: Start with anywhere from three to ten minutes for your first sessions, and build from there. Some dogs will soak it up 24/7 (not really, but it seems like it), while others can only handle small doses at first. Most are somewhere in between, with 20 to 40 minutes being a typical range for a professional dog massage, depending on the dog's size, needs, and attention span.

Frequency of Sessions: This will depend on your dog's health and preferences, on the length of your sessions, the techniques you use, on your stage of learning, and just maybe on your schedule! For these techniques, every day could be fine for many dogs, even multiple times a day, but you'll have to let your dog tell you for sure. For the learning process I would suggest at least once a week to maintain and build on your progress.

After a massage, give your dog a chance to move her body in order to feel and integrate the changes that have happened. Doing stretches with your dog is also helpful for this process of integration. You will find resources on learning stretch exercises at *www.AllAboutAnimalMassage.com.*

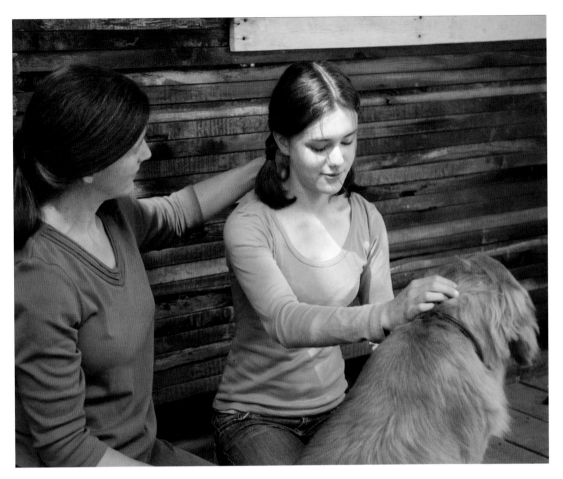

One of the best ways to learn massage is to experience it yourself. In learning how much pressure to use or how fast to apply the strokes, you can use what feels good to your body as a starting point. But remember that your animal may have different preferences, so you do need to listen constantly and be ready to adjust according to her feedback.

Note: Please read all of chapter 6, "Guidelines for Effectiveness and Safety," before practicing any of the following techniques on your dog.

Before practicing each new technique, read the full description along with its Coaching Tips and Anatomy Connection. Trying them out on yourself or a human friend is also a great way to get more feedback on your touch.

Technique 1
Full Body Stroking

Known technically as *effleurage* (pronounced ***eff**-lur-ahge*), this stroke might seem too simple to count as massage, but if you practice with the three coaching tips below, you and your dog will both experience how therapeutic it is. Think especially about the circulatory effects you read about in chapter 3. In addition to being quite relaxing, effleurage is excellent for stimulating circulation. Understanding and visualizing this information clearly will enhance the effects.

You can begin stroking gently either on your dog's face, head and ears, or on his body, but eventually you will cover the whole body from nose to tail to toenails. Most often you will use a full hand contact, but at times maybe fingers, the back of your hand, or a forearm will be preferable, depending on what's comfortable. Use long, rhythmic strokes that connect one region of the body into another. This will enhance your dog's sense of connection and wholeness in his body.

Swelling: Effleurage strokes are often applied in the same direction the coat grows for animals. Against the fur is also fine, however, as long as your dog does not object. If your dog has any swelling anywhere, you can encourage the excess fluids to move back toward the heart, whether this direction is with or against the fur.

> *If your dog's paws are very sensitive and he pulls them away from this stroking, don't worry about it for now. You will help him get over this as you work up to Technique 7, Pleasing the Paws.*

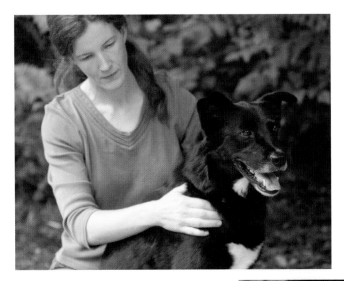

You can begin the massage with your dog sitting or even standing, knowing that as she relaxes she will settle down. Notice a soft hand naturally follows contours of the body.

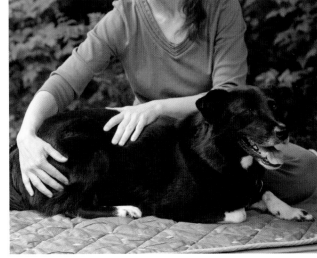

Darcy is beginning to relax and soften her eye. Notice the strokes are connecting the back into the hindquarters and leg.

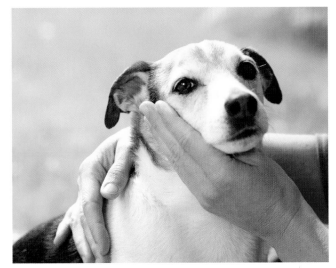

At times you may not have space to use your full hand for the strokes, especially on smaller dogs. Notice my other hand, while not working, is still connected and supportive.

Coaching Tips

1. Breathe. Quietly in and out through your nose. Feel your belly and ribs move gently with your breath. This will help your dog breathe, too.

2. Keep your hands soft, your shoulders relaxed, and your whole body comfortable as much as possible. This will help your dog relax, too.

3. Visualize. Many options here, so feel free to be creative. You can picture the blood flow being stimulated as the vessels relax and dilate (enlarge). You can picture a color or glow spreading slowly across your dog's body, as if you are carefully painting him with your hands. See your dog running and playing with ease, comfort, and joy. Your visualization can be anything, as long as it has these two qualities: it must be positive and it must be about your dog.

Anatomy: The Fascial Web

Effleurage and circulation make a great pair for using the powers of visualization to enhance a massage technique, as discussed above. But since you have already received information on the circulatory system earlier in the book, I will introduce here another huge, important, and wonderful Anatomy Connection that applies equally to all techniques. (Can you tell it's a favorite topic of mine?) Just as the long strokes of effleurage help your dog feel the interconnectedness of his entire body, the following information will help you understand and visualize how thoroughly connected the body really is, even cell to cell.

Fascia, or connective tissue, forms a three-dimensional web of connections throughout the body, changing its form for different jobs as needed by changing the proportions of the molecules that make it up. An analogy, much closer to reality than you might think, would be using flour, sugar, salt, and water (maybe add a few spices?) to make many different foods, depending on the exact recipe. Even bone, for example, is connective tissue with calcium and other minerals added. Layers of connective tissue, including membranes around and within muscles (myofascia), membranes around organs and bones, and the layer of superficial fascia between the skin and underlying tissues, are known collectively as fascia. Tendons and ligaments are actually this very same fascial tissue concentrated into denser forms in order to connect muscle to bone (tendon) and bone to bone (ligament).

It's important to realize that connective tissue is not being used like glue or tape to join separate pieces together, but that the various parts are actually different aspects of one single Whole. *One* spider web spun from *one* strand of silk, so to speak. Thus, every cell in the body has a physical link to every other cell in the body. They are not merely floating side by side in the fluid that is between them.

Though technically not identical terms, *connective tissue* and *fascia* are often used interchangeably. For further fascinating facts about fascia (all the *a*'s following *f*'s should sound the same as you say that), check out the resources at *www.AllAboutAnimalMassage.com*.

Technique 2
Loosening the Legs

Many dogs develop problems with their hips, knees, shoulders, or elbows, so it is very helpful to pay regular attention with massage to these areas, including the whole leg. I find that most dogs are quite receptive to this compression and gentle twist of the muscle tissue below and above the elbows (front legs) and knees (hind legs).

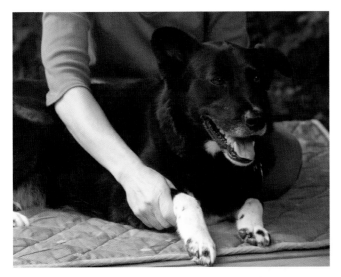

Gently and rhythmically compress (squeeze) your dog's leg. If you listen, your dog will tell you if you're moving too fast or squeezing too hard. You can also add an easy twist while compressing, thinking about the muscle fibers lengthening as they twist slightly around the bone underneath. In addition to lengthening the tissue, you are also helping sticky fibers to separate and pumping fluids through the entire area. You can visualize rinsing out a dirty sponge, and know that the fluids become cleaner each time you repeat the compressions.

My hand is supporting Darcy's leg without gripping. Gripping could make her nervous and more likely to pull away, possibly straining something, and certainly neither relaxing nor trust-building.

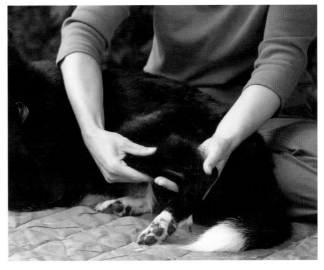

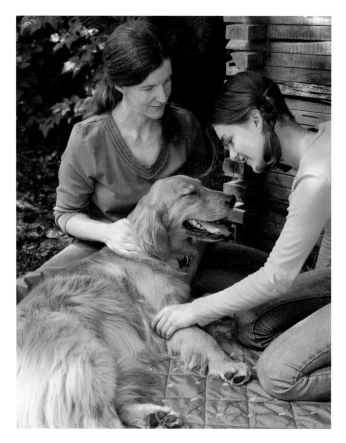

← Hallie is learning to massage dogs. Rosie's face and body language show that Hallie is getting the pressure and speed just right. She is also nicely focused on Rosie's feedback. If Hallie were sitting more comfortably, she could continue massaging for a full session.

→ You can also use two hands to compress and twist. Notice I'm well positioned to avoid needing to lean over or reach too far.

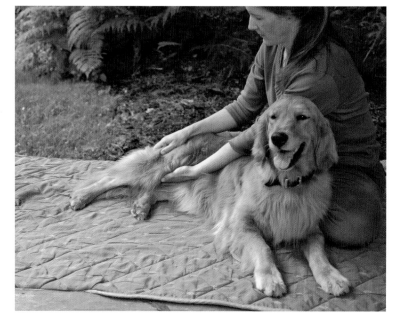

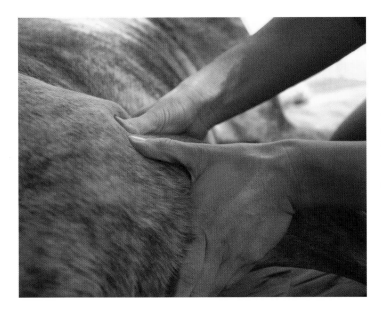

A gental squeeze around Guido's large thigh, without too much pressure on thumbs in this position.

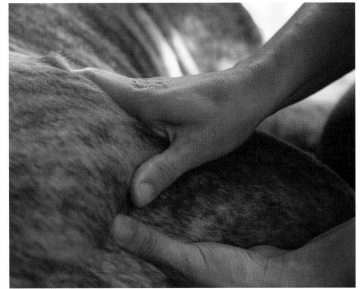

Then rotate the tissue around the bone. In this case the direction my thumbs are moving is from close to his knee back toward his tail, but either direction is fine.

Coaching Tips

1. As you apply the twist, visualize and feel for moving the soft tissue around the bone underneath, but without twisting the bone itself much, which could put a strain on the joints. (If your dog is enjoying it and becoming more relaxed, you can be confident that you are not twisting too much.)

2. An option to the deeper twist effect is to use lighter contact, feeling for just the skin to move sideways over the underlying muscle. This helps free up this more superficial layer (closer to the surface).

Anatomy: Extensors and Flexors

We often hear about flexing muscles, but massage therapists mean something quite different when they talk about flexion. Joints (not muscles) are flexing when the bones are moving closer together, such as when you bend your knee or elbow. Extension is when the joint straightens out again. The muscles that make the joint flex when they shorten (contract) are *flexors*. When the joint flexes and the flexor muscles shorten, the opposing extensor muscles must stretch. Just reach down to touch your toes, bending at your hips (flexing them), and you will feel your hip extensors (the hamstring muscles at the back of your thigh) having to stretch. Likewise, when a joint is fully extended, the flexor muscles must lengthen and stretch. There are other names for movements in more directions (such as rotation, adduction, or circumduction, to name a few), but flexion and extension are the most common.

For every movement that each joint in the body can make, one or more muscles must shorten and others must stretch. When any muscle or group of muscles is tight or glued to other tissue with adhesions, then the joints' movements will be restricted, and the pressures in the joint will be uneven. As you Loosen the Legs, you are massaging the flexors and extensors of your dog's hips, stifles, hocks, shoulders, elbows, wrists, and even all the toes (see Technique 7: Pleasing the Paws), helping to maintain or improve range of motion for the entire leg and the health of all the joints.

Technique 3
Helping the Hips—Tapotement

We already know from part one of this book how important it is to keep joints as healthy and comfortable as we can for full range of motion. So in addition to Loosening the Legs, you can add the technique of tapotement (pronounced *ta-**pote**-ment*) to give extra attention to your dog's hip joints. You can also use tapotement on other areas of the body to stimulate the production of joint fluid, stimulate weak muscles, and increase focus, relaxation, and body awareness.

Tapotement is like gentle drumming. (Or it can be less gentle at times, but for dogs I suggest sticking with gentle.) This percussion stroke creates a drum-like, vibratory effect in the body. The two types of tapotement that are most useful with dogs are tapping and cupping.

Tapping is a light drumming of your fingertips, either all together in a single beat, or one at a time, one after the other, rolling from pinky to index finger. Try each type on your own head right now and feel the difference. Tapping can be used anywhere, even on bony surfaces such as the head.

Cupping is used where there is enough of a flat surface that the cupped shape of your palm can form a pocket of air against the body. The effect of this percussion with the pocket of trapped air makes a nice echo-y, hollow sound effect and sends vibrations deep into the body.

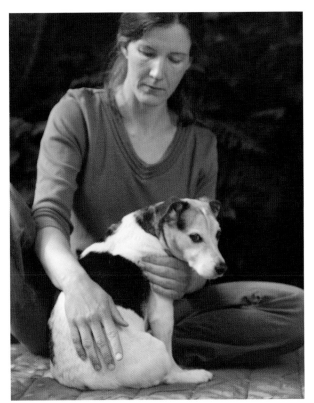

← **Tapping over Gorilla's hip.**

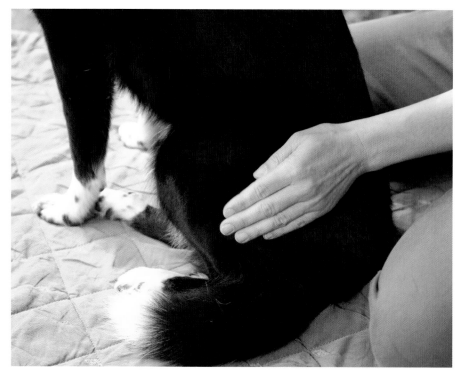

Cupping over Darcy's hip. See also page 61, Balancing the Back, for cupping on Guido's back.

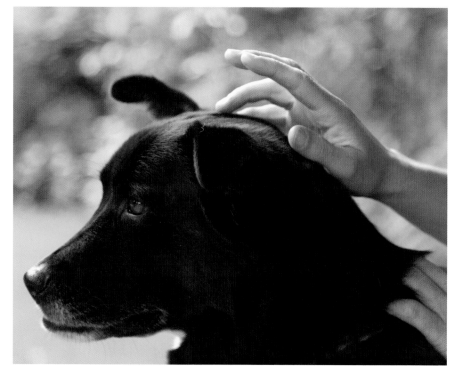

Tapping on Darcy's head.

Coaching Tips

1. For a more pleasant sensation, let your tapotement strokes bounce up off the body more than they fall into it. The heavier stroke without a bounce effect actually deadens some of the vibration you want to create. Feel the difference on your own head (tapping) or thigh (cupping).

2. You can use one or two hands for any type of tapotement. If you use two hands for cupping, use them in an alternating rhythm.

Anatomy: Joint Health

The joints we're most familiar with, including shoulders, hips, elbows, stifles, wrists, hocks, etc., as well as all the vertebral and rib joints along the spine, are all synovial joints (pronounced *sin-oh-vee-al*). This type of joint needs synovial fluid to lubricate the cartilage that covers and cushions the ends of the bones. We know that some dogs stay much more comfortable into their later years than others do. And for any dog, some joints within the body stay much healthier than others. Why is that? Apart from possible genetic or nutritional issues, three main sources of stress to joints are concussion, lack of movement, and unevenness of pressures.

Concussion: The joints are well designed to handle normal concussion, but if there are excessive forces, or if it's repetitive, problems can develop.

Lack of Movement: Movement actually stimulates the joint to produce more synovial fluid *and* makes it thinner and more slippery, like warm, runny oil versus cold, goopy oil. This means the joint is better lubricated, and therefore the cartilage is better protected from damage. When a joint moves less, these benefits don't happen. Lack of movement may involve the whole body, such as with confinement, or a single joint due to tension, pain, injury, or habitual patterns.

Unevenness of Pressures: What if the bones are chronically more compressed on one side of a joint than the other? On the compressed side there's more pressure on the cartilage *and* less room for synovial fluid, so guess where the damage happens to cartilage? And on the other side of the joint, ligaments can be strained where they're being more stretched. Uneven pressures can have many causes, including conformation weaknesses, poor posture, or simply uneven muscle tensions.

Technique 4
Kneading the Neck

For kneading, also known as petrissage (pronounced **pet-ri-sahge**), gently grip and squeeze the muscle tissue along the back and sides of the neck. Then gently lift the soft tissue up away from the underlying bones (neck vertebrae).

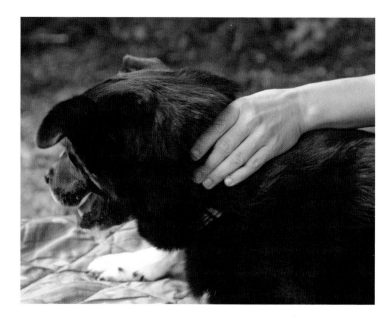

← A relaxed hand ready to start.

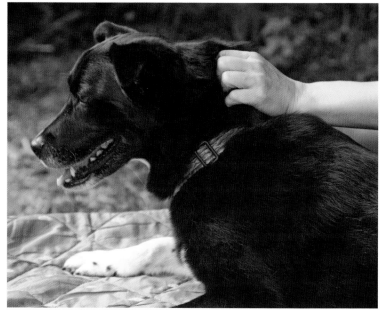

→ The squeeze and lift.

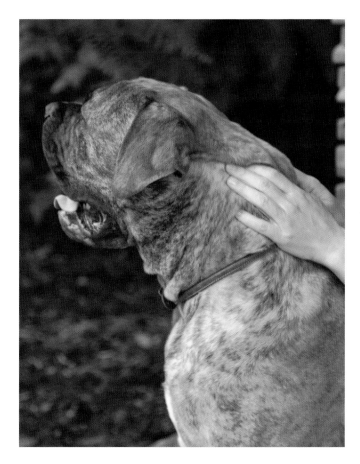

For large dogs like Guido, you may need two hands for this!

Coaching Tips

1. As a general guideline, the deeper the stroke or pressure, the slower you go. For all strokes, you are always feeling for what speed and pressure combination helps the muscles respond and relax without triggering resistance or guarding (see Technique 5 Anatomy: Muscle Guarding). It is not helpful either to you or to your dog to try to push through resistance. Ease off the pressure, slow down (even to stillness at times), and breathe.

2. Expect the first stroke to lift only skin, then the next stroke lifts the most superficial muscle tissue, gradually lifting more and more tissue with each stroke as the layers soften.

Anatomy: Layers—Superficial to Deep

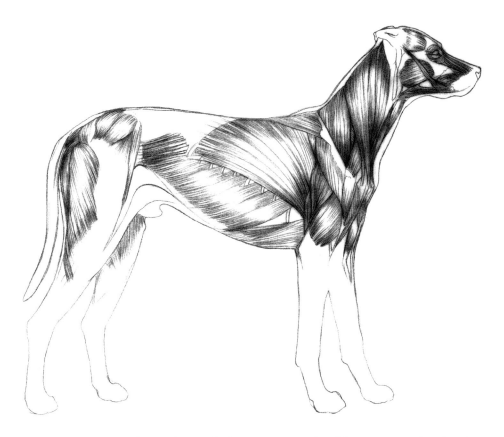

The body has many layers of muscles, with the most superficial lying just under the skin and the deepest located closest to the bones. Each muscle has its own jobs; each usually has a specialty in addition to the other jobs it helps out with. Although we talk about superficial and deep, there are often many more than two layers. Also, a muscle can be deeper near one attachment and more superficial at its other end. As you massage, even if you don't know any of the muscle names, attachments, or layers, you can still practice feeling and imagining the various layers, working lightly at first to warm up, and sensing more of the deeper structures as the muscles relax and soften.

Technique 5
Good Vibrations—Skin and Scapula

It's an understatement to say that vibrations are very powerful. Restrictions can actually melt, in miraculous ways at times, and vibration is one way to add the energy needed for this effect. There are many ways to create a vibration, including the tapotement you've already learned in Helping the Hips. Another way to create vibration is simply to shake the tissue, with as fine (small) and as fast a shake as you can create, so it becomes more like a vibration and less like a shake. You can add a vibration to almost any massage stroke to create more variations.

Try these two examples of vibrating for a wonderful, loosening effect.

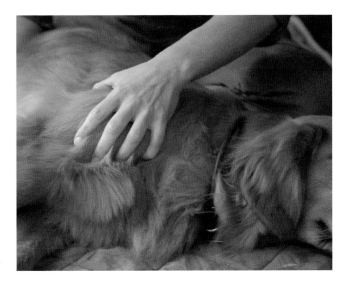

◄
Slightly hook your fingers around the edges of your dog's scapula (shoulder blade), and with very small, fast shakes vibrate the whole shoulder.

➤
You can also vibrate soft tissue only without moving a bone, although when you vibrate the skin and surface muscles along your dog's side, you will also be sending vibrations into the ribs and spine, and even through the whole body.

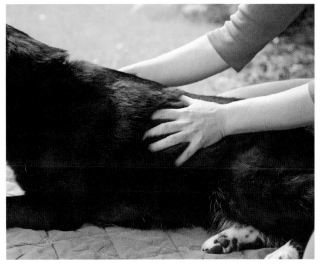

Coaching Tips

1. Imagine the vibrations coming from inside your body, being transmitted through your relaxed arms, and flowing out your hands.

2. Experiment with all possible directions of any vibration movement, side-to-side, up-and-down, in-and-out, diagonal, anything. Listen to what your dog tells you about each variation.

Anatomy: Muscle Guarding

Just as a dog will protect itself if it doesn't feel safe and can't run away, muscles will protect themselves by guarding or contracting, even pushing back at pressure. Often this guarding will happen together with the animal acting worried or defensive, but it is also possible for the animal to be disconnected from part of his body, or to have become used to being stoic or submissive. In this case he may not show signs of negative feedback even though his body itself is guarding. In most cases the state of being disconnected is a result of adaptation, as discussed in chapter 4. Sometimes we adapt to a problem simply by tuning it out, and animals can do this as well, for a certain area or for the whole body. Even if the animal is disconnected, muscles and other tissues can still give you direct feedback, and one of the ways they do this is by guarding. As you help your dog with massage in these areas, he may become more tender or reactive to touch than he was when you started. In some cases this is actually a positive sign of healing as his awareness of and connection to the area returns, or as his inclination to communicate with you grows.

Technique 6
Balancing the Back

For this technique, which is actually a combination of techniques, you will follow the muscles along both sides of the spine. This is a key segment of the Bladder Meridian, more impressively known as the Master Meridian, an energy pathway significant to acupuncture, acupressure, and other forms of bodywork. Try the following variations of applying strokes along these muscles from the top of the shoulders onto the rump. You can do one side of the back at a time or both at once, depending on your dog's position and your preference.

In addition to using effleurage as you did in Full Body Stroking, you can massage these muscles and stimulate the Bladder Meridian in the following ways. See the Anatomy section on page 64 for more information on the meridians.

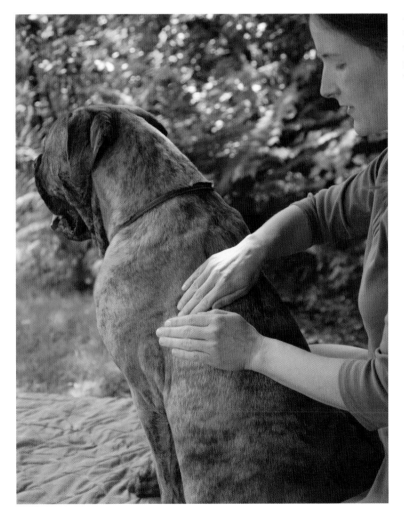

Cupping (tapotement) along the large back muscles. One side at a time will work best for this technique.

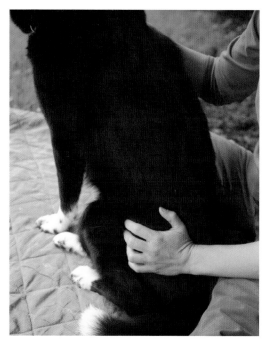

You can compress the soft tissues using the heel of your hand to each side of the spine.

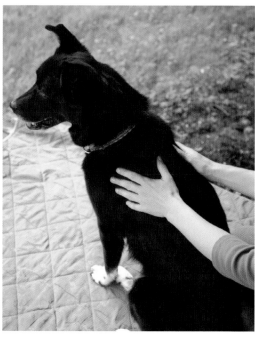

If you use thumbs to compress, keep forearms, wrists, and thumbs nicely aligned.

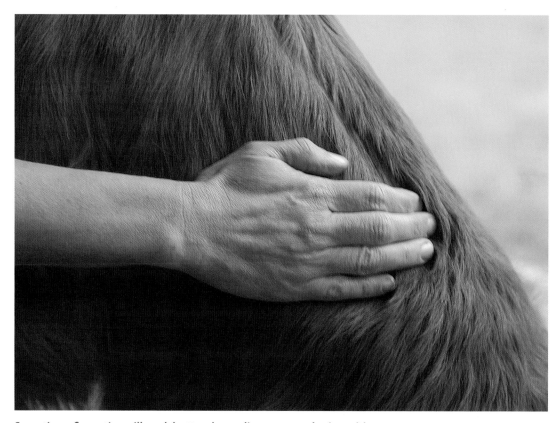

Sometimes fingertips will work better, depending on your dog's position.

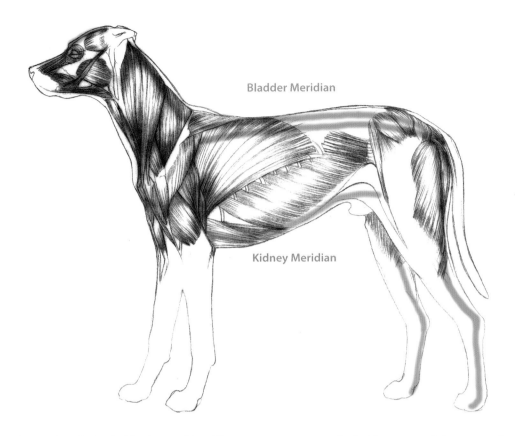

Bladder Meridian

Kidney Meridian

To follow the whole Bladder (Master) Meridian you can start near the inside corners of the eyes and go all the way to your dog's outside toe on the hind paws. The Kidney Meridian is the partner meridian to the Bladder Meridian.

Coaching Tips

1. Try this sequence for each side of the body. First use a long effleurage stroke following the entire length of the Bladder Meridian from between the eyes to the hind paw. Next use one or more varieties of the strokes shown in the photos in this section just along the back and rump. Finally repeat the single, long stroke to reconnect the whole length of the meridian.

2. For the compression varieties shown (heel of hand, thumbs, or fingers), compress in as you exhale and release the pressure as you inhale.

Anatomy: The Meridians

In Traditional Chinese Medicine (TCM) and systems of healing related to it, pathways through the body known as meridians are used in acupressure (with finger pressure) and acupuncture (with needles) for treating a wide range of conditions and symptoms, often with great success. Of the seven pairs making up the major meridians, the Bladder Meridian is recognized as the Master, and its paired partner is the Kidney Meridian. The Bladder Meridian runs from head to toe along the backside of the body. It is no coincidence that this meridian which is known as the Master Meridian also happens to follow the soft tissues alongside what is known as the central nervous system in the West, housed in our spine and skull. It is considered the Master Meridian because points alongside the spine have important connections with all of the other meridians. So as you apply strokes, compressions, or cupping along the Bladder Meridian, bringing your dog's awareness to it, relaxing muscles and stimulating circulation along it, you are indirectly helping to stimulate and balance the energy flow along all the meridians throughout your dog's body.

Technique 7
Pleasing the Paws

This is a natural extension to Loosening the Legs. To prepare your dog now for adding in the following moves, start with leg compressions (and any other techniques you are reviewing as a warm-up today), and work your way from the legs down into the paws. Simply continue the leg compressions all the way down to the paws. If your dog pulls away at any point, relax your hold but stay connected (your hand following any movement of your dog's leg) until the leg relaxes again. Restart the compressions higher up on the leg, and each session work only as far down as your dog can enjoy, knowing that as you repeat this technique over time you will get closer and eventually onto the paws.

If your dog is still not ready for Pleasing the Paws after three to ten sessions of building toward it in this way, don't give up! You can keep at it with this approach, work with a professional, and/or use the resources on the website www.AllAboutAnimalMassage.com to help your progress.

Some forms of bodywork, such as acupressure and reflexology, place great emphasis on fingers and toes, or in this case paws, achieving wonderful benefits for the whole body indirectly through pressures here. Just how these releases are achieved is a bit more mysterious than some other techniques, but this only shows how much we have yet to learn about the body's many connections. Once you experience the profound relaxation from such simple attention, you will know how much your dog can benefit, too.

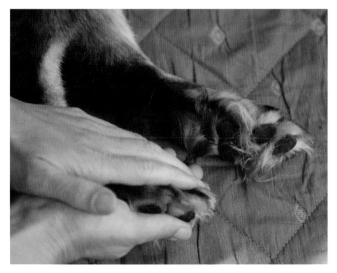

◄
Use two hands with little or no compression if your dog prefers. Holding the paw in this way also promotes relaxation. This and the other variations can help make nail clipping easier, which is important for the health and comfort of your dog's toes, and therefore the rest of the body.

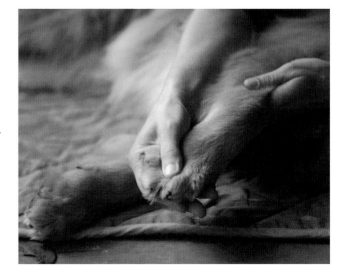

Or you can squeeze each toe, slightly straightening the joints as you compress. Notice the other hand supporting the leg without gripping.

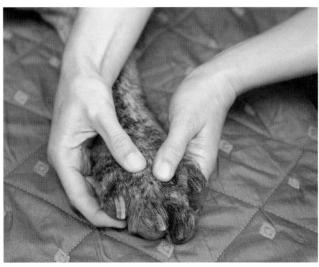

Some paws will take two hands! You can also hold individual toes and move them up and down to further loosen the joints.

Coaching Tips

1. You can avoid resistance in your dog by not giving her anything to resist against. If she pulls her leg away, do not grip or pull back, but simply follow her motion until she relaxes again.

2. You can open your hand so you simply support the leg without holding on to it. Try jostling it gently or repeat the Loosening the Leg compressions higher up, and work again toward the paw.

Anatomy: Lower Limbs

Place your hand palm down on a table, floor, or on the chair beside you. Now lift your wrist so your fingers are still flat but your palm is vertical and in line with your arm, with wrist straight. (You might need to adjust your position to keep everything comfortable.) Your dog walks on his fingers more or less in this way (for the front legs), though the angles of the finger bones are a little different for better shock absorption. What seems a bit like a knee above his front paws is equivalent to our wrist, or carpus. Now for the hind legs. Keep your toes flat on the floor and lift your heels as high as they'll go, as if you're wearing very high-heeled shoes. Your ankle is the same as your dog's hock, and up higher is his knee, or stifle. There is virtually no muscle tissue in these lower limbs from the wrists and hocks down. The movements here are created by the muscles higher up the leg, where you apply the compressions and twists for Loosening the Legs. The tendons of these muscles are very long, reaching all the way down to the toes where they attach into the bones. Any problems in these tendons will be very directly connected to muscle issues higher up.

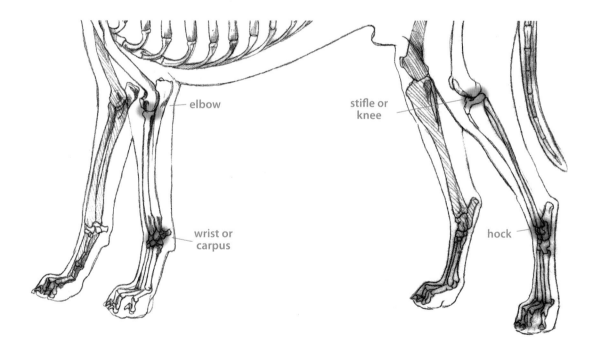

Technique 8
Bony Borders

Whenever I teach animal massage classes, I always emphasize the importance of paying attention to "bony borders," not only the fleshier areas of the body. This is where the muscles (or tendon part of the muscle) are attaching into the bone. There are always multiple structures and tissues overlapping here, with many opportunities to become stressed and adhered to each other: muscle, tendon, membrane around the bone, ligaments, joint capsules, and nerves. Your fingertips are a very useful tool for close attention along bony borders. You can use them to apply rhythmic compressions, small circle motions, or gliding along lines. These same three techniques are useful to find things like adhesions and tender points, and also to help them release.

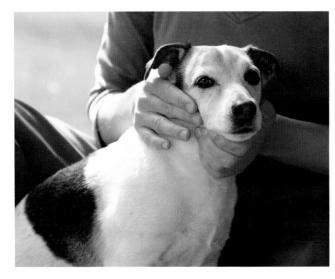

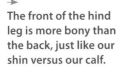

◄
Compressions and small circles along the jaw line are great for those chewing and smiling muscles.

➜
The front of the hind leg is more bony than the back, just like our shin versus our calf.

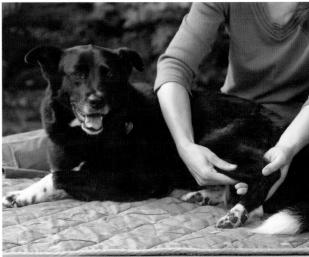

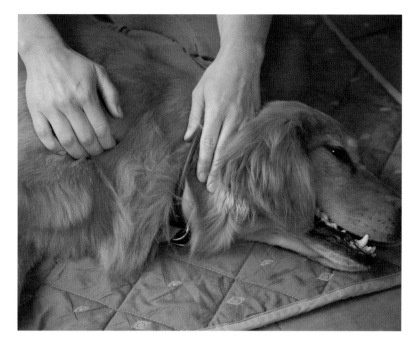

Working along and even curling under the front of the shoulder blade (scapula) is great for loosening many tensions. You're also not far from some of the neck vertebrae here.

Coaching Tips

1. Whenever you use your fingertips, be sure that you do not hyperextend the joints of your fingers. One advantage to using fingertips is that by focusing your contact into a very small area, it takes less pressure to get the same effect. However much pressure you are using, even very light, keep your fingers either quite straight or slightly curved, not hyperextended (not bent at all backward).

2. A nice alternative to fingertips is to use one or more knuckles. This gives you the advantage of a more focused effect. It is a different feel for both you and your dog than using the pads of your fingers, so practice both.

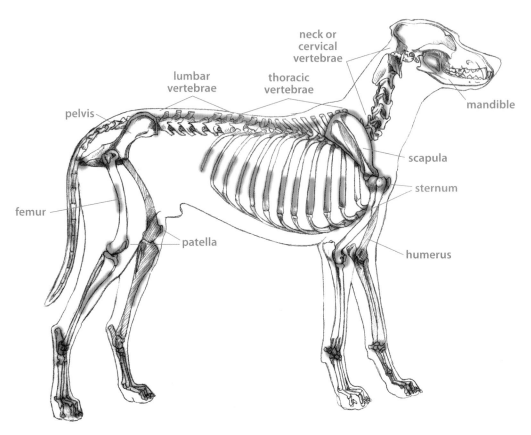

neck or
cervical
vertebrae

lumbar
vertebrae

thoracic
vertebrae

pelvis

mandible

scapula

sternum

femur

patella

humerus

Follow around and along these bony borders in the ways suggested on pages 68 and 69.

Anatomy: The Skeleton

The bones of the skeleton serve many functions. The function we may think of first is that of giving our bodies some "integrity" (remember *tensegrity* from chapter 3?) so that our muscles, skin, blood, and organs aren't just a collapsed blob on the floor. But the bones have several other important jobs. The marrow inside many of the bones produces our blood cells. For some parts of our body, the skull and brain for example, the bones serve as protection for vulnerable organs. They also function as a "bank" for important minerals, including calcium, where extra can be stored until it's borrowed again later when needed.

Here are just a few useful bone names for you to learn to get started.

- **vertebrae:** the small bones that form the spine (singular: vertebra)
- **scapula:** the shoulder blade
- **sternum:** the breastbone
- **humerus:** the upper arm bone
- **femur:** the thigh bone
- **pelvis:** the hip bone (the top of the femur joins it to form the hip joint)
- **patella:** the kneecap
- **mandible:** the lower jaw bone

Technique 9
Immune Boost

With soft, flat fingers, feel gently between the front of the shoulder and the sternum until you have an impression of the most delicate, hollow, or soft-feeling area. Here you will use very light pressure, but also just enough so that as you move your hand gently in circles, the skin moves with your fingers. At the completion of each circle, pause and lighten the pressure even more without losing contact, and imagine and feel for the skin and underlying tissues to rise up and follow your connection. Do about 15 to 30 circles on each side. Longer is fine if your dog especially needs this technique or just plain loves it, but you may get even more benefit for the lymphatic system by repeating 15 to 30 circles at a time several times throughout the session, rather than more all at once.

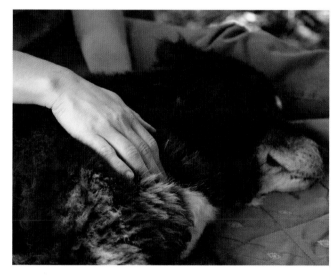

Older dogs will especially relish this, though I have yet to find a dog who doesn't love it.

For smaller dogs there may be room for only a finger pad or two.

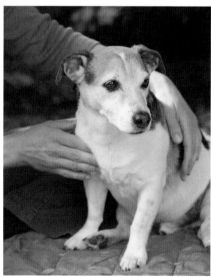

Coaching Tips

1. Visualize the lymphatic fluid like water, now clean and filtered by the body, flowing back into the circulatory system near the heart.

2. This area on the chest is also a powerful calming point. You can often use this immune boost technique to help your dog calm her energy when she doesn't seem ready to relax for other massage techniques.

Anatomy: Lymphatic System

This technique is a perfect example of how one apparently simple move is operating on many levels at once. The top two aspects of anatomy I like to keep in mind when applying this technique are the lymphatic system (almost synonymous with the immune system) and the Kidney Meridian, from the tradition of Eastern modalities such as acupressure and Shiatsu. (See Technique 6 Anatomy: The Meridians, page 64, for more information on the meridian system.) Very briefly, for the lymphatic system, your hand placement is over the area where the filtered lymph fluid has reached the end of its path and is now reentering the bloodstream. As you stimulate the area, you are stimulating this process of lymph vessels emptying fluid into the bloodstream. This creates a siphon-like effect, which draws more lymph into and along its system of pathways. When the lymphatic system is sluggish (slow-moving fluids), it is at a big disadvantage in its job of keeping us healthy, so stimulating the process is a great boost for immune strength. Your hand will also be very close to or even directly over the end point of the Kidney Meridian, also used for strengthening the immune system and a good point for calming energy.

By now you have practiced all nine techniques taught in this chapter, and perhaps a number of variations of them as well. You may even have already begun to experiment with creating your own moves, which is a wonderful urge to follow. Are you noticing how much more awareness and understanding of your dog's body you are developing? And have you experienced any shifts in your relationship and communication yet? There is so much to learn and discover, and you are well on your way along this fulfilling and rewarding path. Congratulations! Now keep on massaging, and come visit us at www.AllAboutAnimalMassage.com to keep on learning.

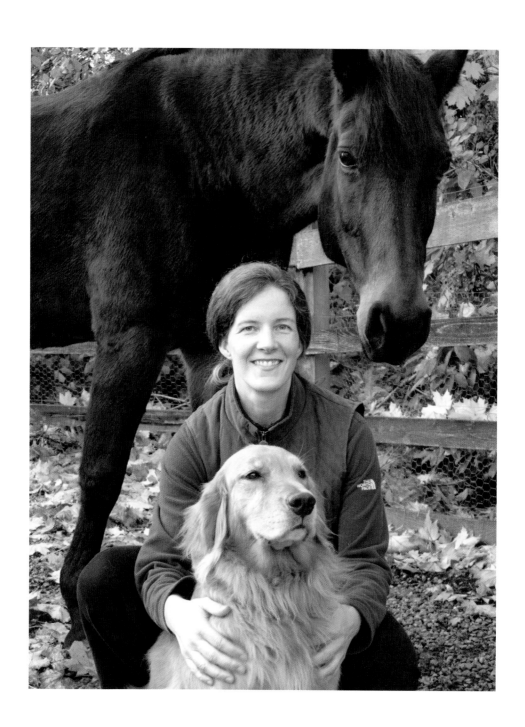

An Invitation

All living beings are literal connections between Earth and Heaven. Earth, in this sense, is the physical, while Heaven is the life force, the soul. As long as there are living things, there is a union between the two. We and our animals are the embodiment of this relationship, and the healthier we are in body, mind, and soul, the stronger that connection is. Taking care of yourself is, therefore, an important commitment that benefits the world, not just yourself.

Also important is to contribute in some way to the health and well-being of others, including the animals in your life, just as you are doing now by learning about animal massage. I have chosen a specific focus for myself that many of you may share. Having spent a number of years volunteering for and eventually as an instructor with therapeutic riding centers, I have a special interest in the well-being of therapy animals. I have a specific vision that all horses serving people in therapeutic programs receive regular bodywork. This would be an important addition to the other forms of appreciation and attention they already receive from their riders, handlers, and care-givers. There are so many ways to contribute, whether by massaging, raising funds, organizing, educating, or inspiring. In fact, in buying this book and anything else from the website, you are already contributing, as a portion of all proceeds are dedicated to promoting and providing massage and bodywork for therapy animals serving nonprofit organizations. Please visit my website *www.AllAboutAnimalMassage.com* for more information.

I hope you have found this book to be a valuable resource, raising your awareness of how the body works and responds to touch, and making the quality of the care you are able to provide the dogs in your life even higher. I also hope you feel and believe, perhaps more than you did before, that you have great power to help the animals you love with massage!

Love,

Megan Ayrault

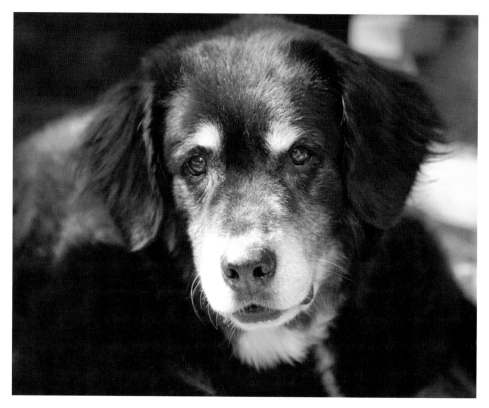

Megan's dog Jessie invites you to check out the All About Animal Massage e-books, teaching more massage techniques, including those especially loved by senior pets.

Glossary

acupressure: use of pressure to stimulate acupoints along meridians to balance the flow of Chi energy

acupuncture: use of needles to stimulate acupoints along meridians to balance the flow of Chi energy

adaptation: changes in a living organism that help it cope with stresses and pressures

adhesion: abnormal binding together of tissues

bodywork: any therapeutic system of touch or manipulation for healing purposes, including massage, acupressure, chiropractic care, yoga, Rolfing, etc.

cartilage: fibrous, elastic tissue acting as a cushion at ends of bones

chiropractic adjustment: manipulation of a subluxated joint, or subluxation, by a chiropractor (see subluxation)

compensation: one or more structures of the body working harder or in a different way than normal in response to dysfunction in another structure or structures

concussion: impact of physical forces into joints and bones

conformation weakness: an aspect of an individual's structure that is more prone to stress and strain in bones, joints, or soft tissues

Craniosacral Therapy (CST): a system of bodywork addressing fascial restrictions and the movement of cerebral spinal fluid within the central nervous system from brain to sacrum (base of spine)

diagnosis: identification of a disease or condition by its symptoms and by diagnostic procedures

edema: excess fluid between cells, swelling

effleurage: a soothing massage stroke that warms surface tissues and stimulates blood flow

endorphins: compounds produced within the body that create a sense of well-being and reduce pain

fascia: a type of connective tissue forming membranes of varied thickness throughout the body

hock: the equivalent of the human ankle, the joint in the hind leg below the stifle

immune system: a combination of mechanisms of the body that work to prevent and fight disease

joint capsule: a tough membrane around the structures of a synovial joint containing the synovial fluid

knots: adhesions in soft tissue that can be felt as fibrous lumps

ligament: connective tissue bands connecting bone to bone

lymph, lymphatic fluid: fluid throughout the body that nourishes cells and transports waste products, white blood cells, and other molecules (some fats and proteins)

lymph nodes: small glands in the lymphatic system that filter lymph fluid and prevent infections from spreading

Manual Lymphatic Drainage: one of several names for a type of massage that focuses on stimulating the movement of lymphatic fluid to reduce edema and support the immune system

modality: within the larger context of bodywork, each distinct type or system of therapeutic touch is a modality. Bodyworkers may be trained in one or multiple modalities.

muscle guarding: when a muscle tenses or holds in order to protect an area or prevent a movement

myofascia: the fascia within and surrounding a muscle (*myo* refers to muscle tissue)

Myofascial Release: may refer to a modality of bodywork in itself or a technique within other modalities. It improves the function and flexibility of fascia (especially, but not limited to, myofascia) by lengthening, hydrating, reducing adhesions, or unwinding. Unwinding is a term describing fascial release and reorganization, including emotional and positional (movement) releases.

palpation: use of feel to assess texture, temperature, tension, tenderness, and range of motion

parasympathetic system: part of the autonomic, or automatic nervous system that triggers rest and relaxation responses in the body

patella: the kneecap

petrissage: variations of massage strokes that compress, knead, and wring muscle tissue, working deeper into the layers beneath the skin

physiology: the study of the functions of living organisms; how structures of the body work

prognosis: a prediction of how a condition or disease will progress

proprioception: the sense of the body's position in space, including the relative positions of different body parts to each other

range of motion: the movement available at any given joint

repetitive stress injury: an injury that results from the cumulative effect of a series of smaller stresses

scapula: the shoulder blade

Shiatsu: (*lit.*, finger pressure), a system of bodywork originating in Japan, based also, historically, on modalities from China; uses a combination of compression massage, acupressure, and stretches

sternum: the breastbone in the center of the chest

stifle: the equivalent of the human knee, the joint in the hind leg below the hip and above the hock

stress point: usually located at the junction between muscle and tendon; an area of stress, pain, and dysfunction that responds well to massage

structural integration: a category of bodywork that uses soft tissue manipulation to realign the skeletal structure for better function and efficiency; includes Rolfing and its offshoots

subluxation: in the context of chiropractic care, a subtle misalignment of a joint that impacts nerves, muscles, and other soft tissue structures

sympathetic nervous system: part of the autonomic, or automatic, nervous system that triggers fight or flight responses in the body

synergistic: when the outcome, or whole, is greater than the sum of the parts

synovial joint: type of joint having a joint capsule containing synovial fluid, which lubricates and nourishes the cartilage of the joint

tapotement: a category of percussive (drum-like) massage strokes

tendon: tissue connecting muscle to bone

tensegrity: a term created to describe a synergistic balance of tension and compression, resulting in "tensional integrity"

toxin: a poisonous substance

trauma: a physical or emotional injury

trigger point: a sensitive point or nodule within a muscle that triggers a pattern of pain when pressure is applied

vertebra (singular), vertebrae (plural): irregularly shaped bones that join together to form the spine, including cervical (neck), thoracic (upper back), lumbar (lower back), sacral (base of spine), and coccygeal (tailbone) vertebrae

www.AllAboutAnimalMassage.com

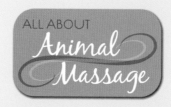

GOOD FOR ANIMALS, GOOD FOR YOU.

Home · About Us · News & Events · Experts · Training · Resources · Store

Welcome to All About Animal Massage!

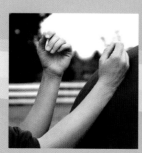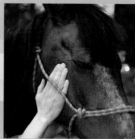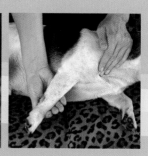

Resources

To continue your education and inspiration, please visit *www.AllAboutAnimalMassage.com* for the following resources:

- Expert Advisory Board

- Free "All About Animal Massage" newsletter

- The "Animal Wellness Network"

- "Ask Megan" Animal Massage Blog

- Recommended books, videos/DVDs, e-books, and other products

- Workshops, webinars, and other events

- Schools offering training and certification

- Links to animal massage-related organizations and websites

- Research and other articles

- Find a professional in your area

- Support massage for therapy animals

- Video clips available for viewing

These many resources provide information and services covering a wide range of animal massage topics and related care, including:

- Massage for cats and other animals, as well as dogs and horses

- Massage for older animals, or those needing extra TLC

- Information on varieties of massage and bodywork

- Animal anatomy

- Animal massage regulations

- Chiropractic care

- FAQs

Below are just a few examples of the many recommended books and videos available in our store at *www.AllAboutAnimalMassage.com*.

Books

Hannay, Pamela. *Shiatsu for Dogs*. London: J.A. Allen, 1998.

Kainer, Robert A., DVM, and McCracken, Thomas O., MS. *Dog Anatomy: A Coloring Atlas*. Jackson, WY: Teton NewMedia, 2003.

Snow, Amy and Zidonis, Nancy. *The Well-Connected Dog: A Guide to Canine Acupressure*. Larkspur, CO: Tallgrass Publishers, LLC, 1999.

Stein, Diane. *Natural Healing for Dogs and Cats*. Freedom, CA: The Crossing Press, 1993.

Videos

Michelin, Lola. *Small Animal Massage Demonstration*. Redmond, WA: Northwest School of Animal Massage, 2006.

Rugaas, Turid. *Calming Signals: What Your Dog Tells You*. Wenatchee, WA: A Dogwise DVD, 2000.

Index

Notes

Notes